STILLNESS TOUCH

UNION OF BODY & LOVE

CHARLES RIDLEY

DYNAMIC STILLNESS PRESS

This book is not intended to replace the services of a licensed health care provider in the diagnosis or treatment of illness or disease. Any application of the material set forth in the following pages is at the reader's discretion and sole responsibility.

ISBN-13: 978-1-7356244-0-2 (paperback)

ISBN-13: 978-1-7356244-1-9 (ebook)

Publisher's Cataloging-in-Publication Data provided by Five Rainbows Cataloging Services
Names: Ridley, Charles, author.
Title: Stillness touch : union of body & love / Charles Ridley.
Description: Morton Grove, IL : Dynamic Stillness Press, 2020. | Includes bibliographical references.
Identifiers: LCCN 2020915766 (print) | ISBN 978-1-73562-440-2 (paperback) | ISBN 978-1-73562-441-9 (ebook)
Subjects: LCSH: Touch--Therapeutic use. | Mind and body therapies. | Consciousness. | Meditation. | Self-actualization (Psychology) | BISAC: BODY, MIND & SPIRIT / Healing / General. | BODY, MIND & SPIRIT / Mindfulness & Meditation. | HEALTH & FITNESS / Alternative Therapies. | SELF-HELP / Spiritual
Classification: LCC RZ999 .R53 2020 (print) | LCC RZ999 (ebook) | DDC 615.8/52--dc23.

Library of Congress Control Number 2020915766

"Caregiver Vulnerabilities to Ethical Misconduct" by Kylea Taylor. Reprinted by permission.
Figure design & creation by Julia Aquino
Content editing by Michaela Sol
Cover design & book layout by Michaela Sol & David R. Sol

Printed in the United States of America
Dynamic Stillness Press is an imprint of Green Tomato Publishing, LLC, Morton Grove, IL, info@greentomatopublishing.com

Stillness Touch: Union of Body & Love/Charles Ridley. —1st ed.
Charles Ridley can be reached at www.DynamicStillness.com

CONTENTS

INTRODUCTION

Laying on of hands for healing has existed for thousands of years in the spiritual traditions. Modern cranial practice began in 1898 when, as a student at the Osteopathic College in Kirksville, Missouri, William Garner Sutherland walked past a skull on display in the college entrance hall. A direct intuition grabbed him that lasted his entire life, as Dr. Sutherland writes, "The thought came, like a bolt from the blue, 'beveled like the gills of a fish,' indicating articular mobility for a respiratory mechanism. That is how the cranial concept came. It is not mine. It never has been." [1]

Even today, medical dogma asserts that no motion exists between the cranial bones; imagine how radical Sutherland's intuition about cranial articular mobility was 122 years ago. He dedicated fifty-five years of study that yielded three types of cranial work. First, Dr. Sutherland introduced biomechanical cranial - a brilliant anatomical structure-function approach, requiring a skillful tactile knowledge of cranial suture architecture. Then, he discovered the cranial rhythmic impulse and functional cranial therapy was born. Here, instead of being guided only by the biomechanical positions of the cranial bones, the cranial wave also guides the functional treatment. In the 1940s, after Dr. Sutherland moved to the California Coast, he realized that the practitioner is not the doer; it is the unerring potency of the Breath of Life that guides a session.

From then on, Sutherland emphasized a non-doing approach to cranial practice, which Dr. Becker later coined biodynamic. A biodynamic session begins when the practitioner realizes a neutral that naturally synchronizes awareness with Primary Respiration as the guiding principle. Primary Respiration contains the embryological power that creates the body, so there is no need to follow the cranial rhythmic impulse; instead, a biodynamic practitioner lets the potency of the stillness that is within the fluid tide and long tide of the Breath of Life be in charge.

Sutherland transmitted his spiritual disposition by writing, "In reading between the lines, we suggest the mental vision through the small end of the microscope followed by the view through the big end of a telescope to observe the material elements disappearing into *endless space.*" [2] Here Dr. Sutherland implies a realization of an infinite non-dual consciousness, which he explicitly etched on his headstone as,

BE STILL AND KNOW

Twenty years later, Adah, his wife, completed the phrase, by etching on her headstone, "I AM." Putting their two sentences together reveals a spiritual transmission of the essence of a biodynamic cranial practice:

BE STILL AND KNOW I AM

The verbiage of the Sutherlands transmission is from the Bible, Psalms 46:10, *Be Still and Know that I Am God*; in the Vedas, I AM is the *Self*, the *Purusha*, or God in man.

> *To know I AM implies a realization of the infinite presence of stillness. Consciousness opens to infinity, everything ceases, and Stillness remains. Gone is the human-centric view, tides disappear, and the biodynamic map dissolves. This is the precious spiritual gift that the Sutherlands gave to us.*

After Dr. Sutherland's death, his protege, Dr. Rollin Becker (1910-1996), introduced Dynamic Stillness, a term derived from Swami Chetanananda's two-volume book that characterizes the principles of Kashmir Shaivism.[3] Dynamic Stillness is the English translation for the realization of a sacred union between Shakti and Shiva. Shiva is the infinite presence of stillness in which the Shakti dwells as the Dynamic Pulse that creates all things. By a dedicated Kashmir Shaivism inner practice, these polar principles unite in the body. Union is by integrating the transpersonal consciousness of I AM, after which the infinite presence of stillness descends into the body. Here, within the cells of the body, dwells the substance of the Holy Grail, a Divine Feminine domain where the sacred marriage ignites a second birth, and we realize that the body is love.

This union of body and love in Christianity is called *enfleshment*.

Dr. Becker realized this, and I believe Dr. Sutherland and his wife Adah also enjoyed this domain. But because the osteopathic profession prohibited a public airing of anything resembling spirituality there is no documentation. Again, a non-doing biodynamic cranial practice awakened in Dr. Sutherland after he experienced that it is the unerring potency of the Breath of

Life that does all the healing, which in 1948 he declared publicly in a single line,

"Allowing the physiological functioning within to manifest its unerring potency, rather than the application of blind force from without."[4]

The Unerring Potency of Stillness Makes the Body

Body is nothing more than emptiness,
emptiness is nothing more than body.[5]

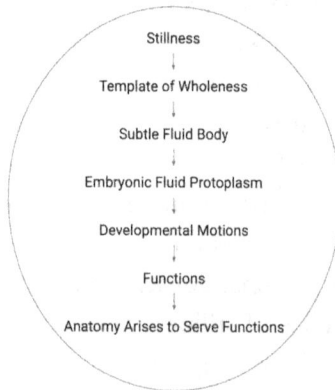

Figure 1. The Unerring Potency of Stillness Makes the Body

Orienting to Anatomy Bypasses Unerring Potency of Stillness

Figure 1: The source of unerring potency is Dynamic Stillness that emanates the template of wholeness to make the body as an indivisible whole unit. The template of wholeness contains the archetypal luminous vibrating geometric patterns that impress a blueprint of the whole body into the *fluid within the fluid* protoplasm of the subtle body. The subsequent biodynamic activity in the embryonic fluids ignites the developmental motions that become the functions, which in turn, creates the anatomy to serve those functions.

Orienting to anatomy by-passes this entire creative whole-making process.[6]

Dr. Sutherland's small circle of osteopaths included Dr. Becker who taught that touching in stillness is neutral, which naturally synchronizes the attention with primary respiration that then guides the touch without doing any treating.

Dynamic Stillness is not an idea; you can realize its uncanny power if you practice what Adah and William Sutherland advised on their gravesite headstones.[7]

"Be Still And Know I AM."

STILLNESS TOUCH: BIODYNAMIC MAP DISSOLVES

Open your heart's door, and let Pure Breath of Love be in charge.

The Dynamic Stillness School offers practitioners a path for the evolution of consciousness. We do not teach biomechanical or functional cranial methods that orient to anatomy, the nervous system, or the cranial wave. Nor do we use biodynamic terms in place of a body-felt experience. We offer a path of development: meditative *Stillness Practices* cultivate a neutral which, amid an inner-body repose while sensing in 'don't know,' presents an opportunity for the *Pure Breath of Love* to take us on a mapless, nameless journey into an unknowable mystery of the body that is in union with love. While in neutral, we dwell in the self-existing heart radiance to sense the qualities that are present without naming them, and we connect to the fulcrum in our pelvis that is united with the Pulse of Mother Earth, which leaves *Pure Breath of Love* in charge.

Stillness Practices prepare you for offering *Stillness Touch* for the evolution of consciousness based on Dr. Sutherland's non-doing. In the book *Stillness*, Chapters 5-9 characterize each cranial enfoldment as an expression of consciousness.

As Dr. Becker taught, the process of transmutation belongs to the Breath of Life, and she does not need our help by doing anything to a client. Instead, we repose in Dynamic Stillness in non-doing, amid a bodily surrender, while yielding our ego to the unerring potency that creates the universe. Yielding our will to *Pure Breath of Love* frees her to suffuse the template of wholeness into every cell of the practitioner and recipient. *Pure Breath of Love* is an alchemical mix of the consciousness of all the elements that form a unique-to-the-practitioner-and-recipient super substance.

Pure Breath of Love is a non-separating matter that lovingly escorts every cell away from inertia and separation and guides it to wholeness that is in a union with The All: this characterizes the essence of a *Stillness Touch* practice.

Realization of *Pure Breath of Love* does not arise until after one's self-sense has disappeared as the doer, and one maintains presence while Dynamic Stillness implodes as inner infinity and *Pure Breath of Love* pours in and takes everything you are.

ANCIENT SPIRITUAL TRADITIONS RECOGNIZE SPIRIT IN MATTER

As quoted above, Dr. Sutherland said that his cranial impulse, "... *is not mine. It never has been."* His precious gift belongs to the whole world backed by thousands of years of practice in spiritual traditions. If offering touch to others as a spiritual practice interests you, let's delve deeper into Dr. Sutherland's biody-namic cranial practice for the evolution of consciousness; we will also explore how the Dynamic Stillness school has evolved the post-biodynamic practice of *Stillness Touch*.

IMPORTANT NOTE: Bear in mind that the sequence of events characterized throughout this book do not occur in the order that I describe them. What unfolds during a *Stillness Touch* session with a living human being cannot be logically mapped and frozen into neat sequences, given the chaotic expression of simultaneous multiple states of consciousness that is our spectral body. A logical map is presented to help the ego feel comfortable amid the extremely messy, uncomfortable, unbearable chaos that is our fully lived spectral reality as a human being. However, at some point, the map has to be put aside *if* we long for union with love.

STILLNESS TOUCH AND THE
EVOLUTION OF CONSCIOUSNESS

A Sutherland-inspired *Stillness Touch* session begins when the *presence of stillness* envelopes your whole inner body space. Stillness emanates primary respiration, the potent embryological force that makes the body, maintains and heals the body, develops our perceptual capacities, and evolves consciousness. By repeated embodied contact with stillness, consciousness *ascends,* which frees it from ego's matter-bound grip of narcissism. Once the wholeness of the body is realized at infinity, consciousness *descends* into the cells and radically awakens them amid a bodily union with love that never ends.[8] Evolution of consciousness involves the ascending and descending current.

ASCENDING AND DESCENDING LIFE CURRENTS
EVOLVE CONSCIOUSNESS

Ascending Current: Evolution of your consciousness begins when the *presence of stillness* envelops your whole-body field and ignites a *fluid presence* inside you. Here, you enjoy the first tidal expression of primary respiration that in biodynamics is called the fluid tide. Your consciousness gradually deepens and expands each time you contact the *fluid presence* until your sense of stillness expands beyond your body into the room to the edge of your known. Meanwhile, there is a profound slowing of primary respiration in which your awareness becomes subtle and expands into a vast *global luminous presence* that is the long tide. This vast breathing field emanates a *global luminous presence of stillness* that not only holds the template of wholeness that makes the body as one unit, it also extends your consciousness to the edge of your known.

Descending Current: After repeated contact with the *vast luminous presence*, you become submerged in an infinite black stillness, and all tidal motions cease. This is called Dynamic Stillness, a domain in which your consciousness spills beyond the edge of the horizon of your known, and the ego, as your sense of a separate self, dissolves. At some point, this infinite *presence of stillness* descends and implodes within the body while consciousness expands beyond all your known reference points.

DYNAMIC STILLNESS IS THE FULCRUM THAT FREES YOUR SPIRIT

When you surrender ego control while reposed in the black space of inner-body infinity, Dynamic Stillness dissolves your ego's separate sense of a self, which permanently frees consciousness from ego's narcissistic grip. Here, in imploded Dynamic Stillness, consciousness crosses the threshold beyond the ego's limitations and becomes universal.

Consciousness radiantly awakens as the *Self* - I AM.

Summary: by repeated contact with the *ascending* current of the *fluid* and *luminous presence,* consciousness gradually becomes free from the ego's narcissistic grip. At Dynamic Stillness, the ego's control over consciousness dissolves, and the I AM is born. After Dynamic Stillness implodes as a *descending current,* it invites *Pure Breath of Love* to suffuse all the cells that unite body, consciousness, and love.

When the inner-body implosion of Dynamic Stillness occurs, that is the fulcrum between the ascending and descending currents that invites into the cells *Pure Breath of Love,* which is a primordial substance that manifests all of creation.

When the Tides Dissolve and the Biodynamic Map is Gone, You Enter the Post-Biodynamic Domain of *Pure Breath of Love*

I remember when this mysterious 'something' appeared during a 2002 Mentor Course in Ithaca, NY.[9] Although no words could convey this mapless realization, the inner-body *presence of still-ness* had the distinct qualities of the tender Mother Love that creates all that is. Here, a Divine Feminine Presence emerged out of an Absolute un-manifest Dynamic Stillness as a singular unit of invisible Wholeness, a 'non-separating' matter that unites everything she touches. From an inner perspective, you sense that *Pure Breath of Love* unites all things. Even though off the biodynamic map, in Kashmir Shaivism *Pure Breath of Love* is called the *Spanda,* which is a *Sacred Tremor* inside every cell that pulses in tandem with the heart's pacemaker that unites you with The All.

When you realize *Pure Breath of Love,* it indicates a sacred marriage - an inner-body union between *Shakti* and *Shiva.* In the East, the feminine principle is called *Shakti,* which is the Dynamic Feminine Force of Love that creates The All. Stillness is the masculine principle, *Shiva,* or Pure Consciousness.

Shiva provides unconditional space for the *dynamism* of *Shakti* to freely express the love that creates all that is.

After *Shakti* and *Shiva* Unite, *Pure Breath of Love* Implodes in Your Cells

As mentioned, this union occurs after Dynamic Stillness implodes inside your body and becomes your perception. Now consciousness begins to integrate as I AM, *Self, Purusha, Shen,* or the *Presence of Stillness,* which are names for primordial consciousness.

Pure Breath of Love is a descending current of utter embodiment that contains an alchemical mix of all prior ascending enfoldments of consciousness that you enjoyed. Again, after your consciousness, as Dynamic Stillness, implodes inside your body, *Pure Breath of Love* suffuses all your cells and radiantly awakens them to consciousness.

NO ME - NO TIDES - NO MAP - NO BIODYNAMICS

At imploded Dynamic Stillness, the tides disappear while *Pure Breath of Love* emerges. However, since *Pure Breath of Love* is off the biodynamic map, once you realize it, your consciousness begins a paradoxical, mapless journey into an unknowable beyond that never ends.[10] You enjoy paradoxical realizations after Primordial Consciousness *descends* to awaken every cell and unites your body with the Tender Mother Love. This is known as enfleshment in the Christian tradition.

The enfleshment of *Pure Breath of Love* is a post-biodynamic realization.

In enfleshment, the classical biodynamic tidal enfoldments disappear and you enter a mapless unknowable journey into primordial love.

AMID AN IMPLOSION OF STILLNESS, THE BOTTOM DROPS OUT TO INFINITY

When Dynamic Stillness implodes in you as an inner body infinity, the bottom drops out while *Pure Breath of Love* utterly suffuses all your cells. In Tibetan Buddhism, this realization is called the *Completion Stage*, the *Great Seal of Perfection*, the *Great Bliss, Dzogchen*, or *Mahamudra*, which bestows the gift of indestructible innocence.[11] It is a great seal of perfection because consciousness has so matured that it is permanently protected by your heart's self-existing radiance that breathes universal love between formless and form. This Unified consciousness reveals that *emptiness is form and form is emptiness*, which is known as the *Prajnaparamita* in Buddhism.

With the realization of *Pure Breath of Love*, a permanent protective seal of Dynamic Stillness suffuses your every cell and unites body, consciousness, and love.

This mirrors the Sutherlands' final advice: Be Still And Know I AM.

A PARADOXICAL STATE - THE PLEROMA

As mentioned, *Pure Breath of Love* combines all your prior realized states of consciousness and unites them as one. Here, all tidal frequencies mix in various combinations to form a single alchemical super substance that powers the unique evolution of your consciousness. A fundamental characteristic of *Pure Breath of Love* is the presence of a paradoxical state: all the qualities of the tides, the elements, and states of consciousness are present, yet you can discern no single quality. Jung calls this the *Pleroma*, a gnostic term that describes the spiritual universe as the abode of God that consists of the totality of the divine powers and emanations.[12] Even amid the presence of *Pleroma*, oddly enough, your prevalent sense of *Pure Breath of Love* is a whole-body, all-cell, pulse that is in tandem with your heartbeat.

Every place you touch is the pulse of *Pure Breath of Love*

EMBODIED MEDITATION CULTIVATES DEPTH

The Embodied Path of Meditation Summarized: When you begin to meditate daily, your presence dips in and out of the *ascending current* of consciousness (fluid and long tide), which gradually expands your awareness, elevating it beyond narcissistic ego control. When your presence attends to the ascending current, it acclimates you to the archetypal power of I AM, or the *Self*. Eventually, the ego's control over consciousness dissolves, which liberates the emergent *Self*. The next stage of meditation cultivates the inner depth of I AM that inwardly concentrates to a small point, implodes, and descends as an infinite *presence of stillness* that dwells inside the body - *if* you dare to surrender and let it happen. Your sense I AM dissolves amid infinite imploded stillness; you may panic here because you have no idea what is happening. Also, amid the ego's dissolution into the *presence of stillness*, your three main soul forces - *thinking, feeling, will* - split apart and you temporarily lose 'I' consciousness. Only after you pop out of the infinite black inner-body stillness do you know that 'something' happened. However, after periodic dips in and out of imploded Dynamic Stillness, your presence can remain awake therein, and your *presence of stillness* becomes unwavering, which marks when Dynamic Stillness, as I AM, becomes your consciousness.

After acclimating to I AM *as* your consciousness, it repeatedly implodes in your inner body space as Pure Consciousness that is the *Self*, and integration begins to dissolve the sense that this is an exalted state; rather it is normal. From now on, you enjoy a continuous indwelling *presence of stillness*, or Dynamic Stillness, that dissolves the notion of an inner and outer infinity because you realize they are one. Then, at some point, inside the imploded *presence of stillness*, all the tidal forces, the consciousness in the elements, and its corollary states gather and rush into your infinite inner space while *Pure Breath of Love* emerges therein. Here you can sense the presence of the Tender Mother Love, which indicates the realization of the sacred marriage between *Shiva* and *Shakti* by which Pure Consciousness and Love become one inside you. These words do not come close to this life-changing inner event, but words are all we have to characterize the fruits of daily meditation.

PURE BREATH OF LOVE'S NON-SEPARATING SUBSTANCE IGNITES A SECOND BIRTH

Pure Breath of Love is a non-separating super substance and everything she touches becomes whole. Like an invisible glue, *Pure Breath of Love* utterly suffuses every cell, awakening them with the Radiance of Love, which is the Divine Feminine principle that unifies all things. This is the same alchemy that powers embryogenesis, which from two cells, creates a fifty trillion-celled human being in nine months. In an adult, *Pure Breath of Love* is the alchemical substance that ignites in you a second birth in which your consciousness enjoys an utter bodily union with all that is. Many spiritual traditions teach that a regular spiritual practice ignites a second birth. Perhaps A.T. Still, the founder of osteopathy, understood this when he said the body is the second placenta.

Pure Breath of Love evolves you beyond the recoils of the ego that began after you suffered the *Core Erotic Wound,* which is the most painful event in your life that formed your personality.[13] After being suffused by *Pure Breath of Love*, you realize that all aspects of your spectral human-beingness are in a body-felt union with The All.

Again, *Pure Breath of Love* is a unique-to-you alchemical mix of all of your states of consciousness that suffuse your cells and bestow a felt-sense of wholeness. I used the analogy of a cake mix during a Harbin Springs Initiatory Class in 2005.

The basic cake ingredients are flour, milk, eggs, sweetener, fat, and baking powder. Then, depending on what kind of cake you're making, other ingredients make the cake chocolate, vanilla, or carrot. So *Pure Breath of Love*, like a cake mix, contains all the enfoldments of consciousness that are necessary for your evolution. This alchemical mix is based on other unique ingredients, such as what Buddhists call the 'givenness' of your *Core Erotic Wound*, your biography, and history.

The unique alchemical mix of *Pure Breath of Love* unravels all limitations created by your past traumas, and alchemically transmutes them one by one, which is the process that makes you whole.

At this point, *Pure Breath of Love* suffuses all your cells and radiantly awakens them amid a sensuous body-felt-connection with everything. Unified consciousness replaces a controlling ego that objectifies and separates consciousness into discrete events by naming them. Here, in *Pure Breath of Love*, there are no perceivable stages of separation, your only sense is an utter bodily union with The All.

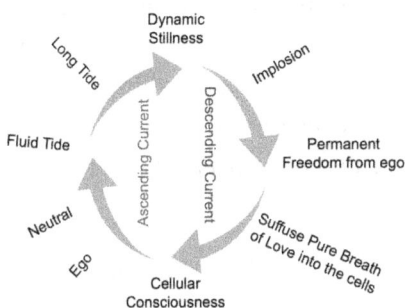

Figure 2. Summary of the Realizations Along Your Meditative Journey

IT TAKES COURAGE OF HEART TO KNOW THYSELF

One challenge, while all qualities and states suffuse your inner body, is to maintain a steady *presence* while *Pure Breath of Love* unrelentingly brings all the separate aspects of your shadow back home to love. It is dreadfully uncomfortable to face all the habitual recoils from love that arise due to the *Core Wounds.* The recoils are in the armor of the body's flesh, in the gelled ground substance, there is electrostatic charge, painful memories, shock, and much more.[14]

Being present to *what is* dissolves the recoils.

It is challenging to remain present to the unbearable discomfort without resistance, yet we have the *Stillness Practices* to daily engage to gradually bodily navigate the inner territory and remain present amid any intensity, intimacy, and paradox.

Our fundamental practice is a turning inward of attention to repose in an unwavering presence. This fortifies us to bear the uncomfortable whole-making process while *Pure Breath of Love* transmutes everything in us that recoils from love. We gradually

9

cultivate a capacity to be with what arises - *as it is* - no matter how uncomfortable, intense, intimate, or paradoxical it feels. *Pure Breath of Love* asks for every skill we have, plus a little more. Yet once we surrender everything we are to love, and we allow love to suffuse every cell in our flesh, there will be zero difference between *Pure Breath of Love* and our body.

WHEN THE BODY IS SUFFUSED BY PURE CONSCIOUSNESS AND LOVE IT IS CRIATURA

Criatura is when the body enjoys its full spectral glory; here are ways to characterize it:

- The body is a subtle infinite shimmering consciousness that emanates love.
- Body is an infinite web of sensuous consciousness.
- Body is the self-existing radiance of the heart united with *Eros* in the pelvis that emanates an infinite tonal web of sensuous consciousness and love.

The self-existing radiance of your heart is the wisdom that makes your body, maintains your body, heals your body, develops your perceptual capacities, evolves your consciousness, and unites your body with love, which culminates in enfleshment.

IN ENFLESHMENT, LOVE IS IN CHARGE

> The body is nothing more than emptiness, emptiness is nothing more than the body. The body is empty, and emptiness is exactly body.[15]

When love moves mind, body, speech, and your will as a whole unit, your whole being seamlessly expresses love. The ego never goes away, and it will continue to complain, resist, and recoil from love; yet, its antics have zero effect because the ego has no power over *Pure Breath of Love*. The power game is over for the ego. Neither its strategies of separation - by objectification, thoughts, stories, emotions, or acts of physical and psychological recoil - can thwart *Pure Breath of Love's* process of whole-making. The ego will continue as long as we are alive. However, if we can trust enough to yield the ego to the benevolence of love, rather than being an adversarial source of our suffering, ego's strategies become entertaining. At the end stages of integration, the ego becomes supportive.

> We not only belong to love but also love belongs to us. It is a two-way evolutionary process in which we co-evolve with love as one unit.

As noted, the enfleshment of *Pure Breath of Love* marks the beginning of the post-biodynamic practice of *Stillness Touch*. This journey into love, as a series of endless realizations of wholeness, awaits you at the Dynamic Stillness School. Can you see that once you have enfleshed *Pure Breath of Love* that you enter a post-biodynamic journey into love? There are no tides, no maps, and no exalted stages, and we enter this post-biodynamic domain as an ordinary human being.

THE REALIZATION OF PURE BREATH OF LOVE ENDS EGO'S ILLUSION OF SEPARATION

In review, *Pure Breath of Love* combines all enfoldments as one: the cranial wave, which is a pre-biodynamic enfoldment that is the holographic record of your past; the biodynamic enfoldments include the fluid tide as 'the given' in the present, and the vast luminous space of long tide, which is your future potential as the *Self*.

CHARACTERISTIC OF PURE BREATH OF LOVE

Pure Breath of Love is always accompanied by the *presence of stillness* as a permanent seal of imploded infinite black emptiness that is Dynamic Stillness, or Pure Consciousness. The seal of Dynamic Stillness permanently protects the potency of the Divine Feminine principle. Amid her unimpeded potency, she can ignite eternal change while maintaining an exact alchemical mix of all the ingredients of consciousness that are needed for the evolution of consciousness for each person moment by moment.

When we realize *Pure Breath of Love*, it ignites an all-cell, whole-body, universal pulse of *Spanda* that is synchronized with the heartbeat. The presence of *Spanda* indicates an inner union between the self-existing radiance of the heart and *Eros* in the pelvis. This inner body union combines Pure Consciousness and Universal Love. *Pure Breath of Love* emanates from all cells and expands to infinity; while simultaneously from infinity it implodes into all the cells and emanates a renewed superradiance of love in your inner body space. Your radiant heart, your *Eros* suffused pelvic heart, the Gaia Heart, and the Universal Heart pulse as One Heart in tandem with your heartbeat.

Your actual sensual perceptions are a combination of all the components below:

- After your heart's self-existing radiance unites with the sensuous *Eros* in the pelvis, Dynamic Stillness implodes inside the body and *Pure Breath of Love* suffuses all your cells. You sense every cell and all fluids sensuously pulse the superradiance of love that erotically unites you with everything.

- You sense *Spanda* as a whole-body all-cell pulse that is

in tandem with your heartbeat. The potency of the pulse continues to expand and strengthen unimpeded by any power. When the pulse periodically evaporates in Dynamic Stillness, your awareness may disappear. When it returns, your consciousness is ordered more coherently and radiantly awake as the *presence of stillness*.

- You intuitively apprehend *Pure Breath of Love*'s pulse as an alchemical mix of all qualities of consciousness and tidal expressions that are one, all of which are sealed inside an imploded inner-body *presence of stillness* - as Dynamic Stillness.

- You sense that your heart's radiant field of *presence* rhythmically expands, strengthens, and then dissipates in intensity. The pulse continues to expand, strengthen, dissipate, and then your heart radiance periodically dips into Dynamic Stillness, and your consciousness disappears while it implodes as Pure Consciousness inside the body's cells. This cellular inner infinity emanates a vast, radiant, *presence of stillness* that unites outer and inner infinity until they become indistinguishable.

- Powerful ignitions occur when your heart radiance disappears into the infinite black Dynamic Stillness.

- At a point beyond the infinite expansion of your heart field, it is as though Dynamic Stillness creates a vacuum at the SA Node that causes its great vastness to implode, rush into the heart and create an inner infinity in the body that becomes the permanent protective seal of Dynamic Stillness.

- When Dynamic Stillness implodes in the body as an inner body infinity, it becomes a 'great seal of protection' for *Pure Breath of Love* that emerges as an alchemical mix of all tidal frequencies of consciousness. Love pulses as a superradiance that suffuses all cells in tandem with the pulse of the SA Node.

- Once the all cell whole-body pulse of *Pure Breath of Love* arises, the *Sacred Pulse* is sensed every place you touch on the body.

STILLNESS TOUCH: A TOUR OF LOVE

Stillness Touch is a post-biodynamic journey of mutuality, and as is always the case during a session, the recipient's subtle body is omniscient. Before touching, a practitioner engages her inner *Stillness Practices*, which also prepares the recipient to openly receive the session, which they feel like a sense of relaxation and trust.

Here are comments from recipients describing a *Stillness Touch* session:

"While my practitioner inwardly prepares, I can feel my flesh soften, and my body sinks on the table into deep relaxation. I feel my practitioner approach me quietly, and she alights her hands on my body. I sense that the qualities of stillness guide her touch because she rests her hands on me without doing anything. I can barely tell she is touching me: it feels as though her hands and my flesh are the same and all I sense is the *presence of stillness*. My subtle body intuitively knows my practitioner has no plan, no goal, and no expectations for any movement patterns to arise in me. Her touch evokes in me a feeling of freedom, and I easily relax because I can trust both the practitioner and the process. I can repose and surrender my whole body that is breathing inwardly as a single, whole unit in an elegant fluid ebb and flow.

I can sense a more subtle inner breathing that wells and builds in strength for a steady 12 seconds, and then it recedes and softens for 12 seconds, which moves every aspect of my body as a whole, like how the sea moves seaweed. The power in this elegant living breathing fluid field gathers all my body's chaotic areas and self-organizes them until they express a harmonious fluid motion of wholeness. I feel re-connected to myself and nature, the way I was as a young child, which evokes in me a sense of belonging and of having returned to my original state before any wounding occurred. After some time, this process culminates and becomes a whole-body, global stillness.

While global stillness grows in potency, it expands my body consciousness that becomes a subtle vast radiance that hovers on the horizon at the edge of my known. My vast radiant body breathes an extremely delicate in-breath that wells, expands, and intensifies for nearly one minute, and then the radiance recedes and softens as an out-breath for a minute. Inside this luminous vastness, I 'see' brilliantly colored geometric shapes that emit ecstatic tones that I 'hear.' Yet, it is not with physical eyes, ears, or senses that I realize this. My whole body seems to become a sense organ that is in touch with everything. Amid these luminous colorful tones and geometric shapes, my perception inverts and shifts from being the one who sees to the one who is seen by a gentle Radiant Presence that unconditionally loves me exactly as I am.

My body is a vast field of stillness that is radiantly present by which I sense everything about myself, including my horrifying core wounds that created the most self-dreaded aspects of my shadow. And yet, since I feel loved just as I am, I can accept myself, and I have the strength of will to feel the full intensity of my shadow. Then my Radiant Presence intensifies and expands and becomes my awareness. Suddenly, my awareness spills over the edge of my known into a black infinity of stillness.

The black infinity of stillness within me is nothing. I have no self-sense, no thoughts, no feelings, no emotions, no memory, no time, and no subtle breathing consciousness. It is all cessation within infinite black space. Cessation seems to continue indefinitely. Then, suddenly, I feel my consciousness is magnetically pulled down, as though I am being forced through the eye of a needle, or a tiny funnel that concentrates my awareness to an infinitesimal point. Then the bottom drops out through my pelvis, and my awareness implodes inside my body and becomes an inner infinity. Infinite black stillness is inside me, and suddenly all the previously realized qualities of my consciousness combine with the imploded black stillness.

This mix includes everything: my life history, my shadow, the *Core Wound*, the fluid flow, the vast luminous radiant presence, and infinite black stillness. This mysterious super-radiant fluidic 'something' unites all that I am with all that is. I feel united with everything, and all of it is love. I sense the super-radiant substance suffuse my every cell with love that pulses with my heartbeat. I have come home to the tender Love of the Mother. My body and love are one, and love is all that is. I feel utterly submerged in this ocean of love for some time, and then I realize that the practitioner is no longer touching me. My session felt like an eternity. When I open my eyes, I feel entirely different, and yet paradoxically, I am the same."

The above inner-body tour of love traverses the classical biodynamic *ascending* map that is the fluid tide, the long tide, and Dynamic Stillness. Then, with the *descent* of consciousness into the cells due to the implosion of Dynamic Stillness, an inner infinity is established within the body, and the session enters a mapless post-biodynamic journey of *Pure Breath of Love*. When every cell is suffused by *Pure Breath of Love*, the practitioner and recipient's heart field is tender, infinite, open, and omniscient.

When a practitioner offers neutral touch, it naturally transmits the *ascending* Breath of Life current to a recipient. However, participation in a post-biodynamic *Stillness Touch* session occurs after the practitioner's consciousness *descends*, amid an inner body implosion of Dynamic Stillness in which pours *Pure Breath of Love*. After this event, the practitioner is unshakably centered in the *presence of stillness*, united with the heart's self-existing radiance at the SA node, inwardly reposed in *Eros* at the pelvis, firmly rooted in the core Heart of the Mother Earth, amid an utter inner body union with pure consciousness and the love of the whole. These realizations are not possible without the practitioner neutral that we will now explore in-depth.

2

CULTIVATING NEUTRAL IS
ESSENTIAL TO STILLNESS TOUCH

People don't understand that the hardest thing is to do something that is actually close to nothing. It demands all of you because there is no story anymore to tell, there are no objects to hide behind, there's nothing, just pure presence.[16]

Consciousness evolves when we repose in neutral, which by definition, means be still. When touching, we do not objectify, evaluate the nervous system's motions, or orient to anatomy to relieve symptoms in a recipient. In a neutral, all we 'do' is to sense within our inner body space. Our inner-body wisdom already resonates with the creative power of the Breath of Life that expresses the template of the Whole. In neutral, we naturally entrain with the recipient's whole body while we are touching them. Dr. Rollin Becker tells us that by reposing in neutral, our inner-body stillness silently communicates with the stillness inside the recipient.

THE SILENT INQUIRY OF THE BODY

When a practitioner is neutral, touch naturally transmits still-ness to a recipient, which prepares them to relax, surrender, and yield the controlling strategies of their ego to *Pure Breath of Love.* When the recipient is neutral, the nervous system no longer controls the recipient's body during the session. Engaging the *Stillness Practice* before touching liberates the invisible embryological developmental forces that are present in the recipient. These forces emerge as an invisible template of wholeness, which you sense as the motion that is present. When a recipient inwardly senses these hidden life forces, she has an opportunity to surrender to them. Without using words, a recipient naturally yields to the Breath of Life; however, when a neutral deepens into a realization of *Pure Breath of Love,* a recip-ient may say to love:

Take me as much as you give yourself to me.

This degree of surrender can only occur when a practitioner is not objectifying a recipient, which means we do not separate the recipient from us, making them an 'other' that we treat to relieve symptoms. Therefore, we refrain from 'doing to' them. *Stillness Touch* is never oriented to the nervous system, to anatomy, to the cranial wave, the tides, or to relieve symptoms. We do not name or tell a client about motions that we think are happening, or are "supposed" to happen. Instead, we repose inwardly in the *presence of stillness* without expectations. Reposing in the innocence of, 'don't know' leaves the recipient free to relax and trust because she senses an empowering message, "I can relax, trust, and surrender." What allows this to happen is the recipient senses that the practitioner "is not a know-it-all and will not mess with my process." You may recall that the recipient's subtle body is omniscient and senses a practitioner's motives.

The Breath of Life freely operates *only* when I am reposed in a state of non-doing. Neutral works like a physics equation: the degree that I 'help' the Breath of Life creates the same amount of efference, which repels the potency until it withdraws from my body-felt experience. Have you ever felt that a practitioner's 'help' during a session hindered your process?

> The highest compliment I can receive is when a recipient says, "I could feel *presence*, but you were not in the way, interfering with my process."

As medically oriented practitioners, we are trained to assume the egoic disposition of, "I am the intermediary between God and the client," so naturally I want to help the Breath of Life by meddling with the client's process. Although this is well-intentioned, I am interfering with the recipients' already ongoing whole-making biodynamic process.

> One of the most challenging points to get across in biodynamics is the practitioner does not have to "do" anything except be still in neutrality.

When you can be still and do nothing, while you touch a recipient, that quality of neutral liberates the template of wholeness that holds the invisible blueprint forces that create an optimal function in the fluids. Then the form, or anatomy, arises to serve the function of health. Reposing in stillness is essential, because inside each bone, each organ, each cell, and everything else in creation there is a fulcrum, a center point of stillness around which formative forces organize the fractal patterns of life that create the function, which, in turn, makes the form. The fulcrum of stillness is in the center as a column of stillness. The destructive forces of chaos are at the outer edge and as you move toward the center, the midline, it becomes increasingly less chaotic until you reach stillness in the core. Healthy fulcra are moving points of stillness that freely flow to serve the function that in turn, creates anatomy. In contrast, inertial fulcra repeat static patterns that drain life force from the body as a destructive death-dealing force.

Stuck patterns of inertia repeat in us in many ways; for example, we exhibit annoying behaviors, or we feel tortured by recurrent thoughts, feelings, emotions, memories, and stories, right? When our patterns repeat, we may say to ourselves, "there's my emotional reactivity acting up again even though I know better!" And on it goes that the recurrent inertial patterns drain our life force to feed the repetitive motions that trap awareness, so inertia has its way with us because our will is too weak to overcome our stuck patterns. By analogy, inertia is a parasite that drains the life forces of health from the body, which weakens our will and leaves us stuck in repetitive patterns that hinder our evolution, and we remain on a downward spiral toward death.

When we suffer from chronic inertia, it compromises our whole system: it diminishes immunity, health, thinking, cognition, emotional vitality, and learning. Our presence waivers and our strength of will weakens. Inertia so drains the life force from our will, that we become powerless and unable to muster the presence required to face our uncomfortable shadow issues that open us to love.

IF YOU DESIRE TO REALIZE PURE BREATH OF LOVE: FACE YOUR SHADOW

Practically speaking, when inertia prevails, the nervous system and ego control the body and its functions. Ego takes charge because we have no contact with the potent forces of life, which diminishes our strength of will. The ego misuses the body's source potency of life, while the nervous system maintains the inertial patterns. This process continues when we obey ego's dictates, leaving our consciousness under nervous system control, which makes it impossible to realize the body's spectral wholeness. If the body becomes overloaded with inertia, the death forces prevail, and life will end.

Given the above, would you rather orient to the nervous system during a *Stillness Touch* session, or yield to the *Pure Breath of Love* and let it be in charge?

> Recall that Becker characterized the neutral as the moment the body is no longer under the control of the nervous system.

I realize that some practitioners may feel stuck in a symptom relief practice; functional work is an excellent medical model approach that I practiced for 20 years. In functional work, we orient to the nervous system and its cranial rhythmic impulse to evaluate function. Then with intention, we move the inertial patterns around in the body, yet have you noticed that there is no overall change in the amount of inertia in a client's body? If you feel trapped in this type of symptom treatment, the way out is to let the *presence of stillness* in the Breath of Life transmute inertial fulcra into living fractals and watch healing naturally occur. As soon as Dr. Sutherland observed and verified this 'uncanny' process, he stopped practicing functional work, saying, "You don't even have to test the sphenobasilar joint." [17]

In contrast to the complexities of functional work, your non-doing practice is simple. In essence, you orient awareness inward, maintain a *presence of stillness* inside you, while you sense the inner body qualities exactly as they arise. You are immersing in the *presence of stillness* while you sense the qualities in your inner body without efference. Your attention is free to move with the fractal motions of the Breath of Life. When attention is free, the stuck, efferent behaviors resolve because your attention is synchronized with the Breath of Life that takes charge of the session. If you repose inwardly with free attention, your awareness moves like a sailboat with the wind and water currents of the Breath of Life.

When we are neutral, we can sense Dr. Sutherland's automatic shifting fulcra that he likened to seaweed that moves with the ebb and flow of the ocean's currents. I prefer to call them *free-flowing fulcra* because that is their body felt-sense. We cannot make a neutral happen; it arises spontaneously. Recall that the beginning of a neutral is when you sense a whole-body stillness that suffuses levity therein. With our presence, we sense buoyancy free the inertia in the body and transmute it to fractal motion. Fractal motion expresses ever-changing qualities of health and wholeness as it arises from the potency of the Breath of Life.

ORIENTING TO ANATOMY IS NOT NEUTRAL

Orienting to the nervous system and anatomy is an anti-neutral act that traps our consciousness in the periphery amid ever-repeating inertial patterns that react to stress. Why do we tolerate inertia, when it bestows 'life as suffering?'

I received a letter from an osteopath who characterized the essence of Sutherland's biodynamics the way that cranial osteopaths practice it. He said that during his postgraduate biodynamic osteopath classes in Holland and Belgium between 2003 and 2011, Dr. James Jealous taught him from day one, very clearly, that all aspects of the healing process come from the Breath of Life by primary respiration, through neutral.

It is by being neutral that we synchronize with the Breath of Life, the osteopath told me. He also said, what I teach is not different from what Dr. Jealous taught them, and it is in perfect alignment with the teachings of Sutherland: no forces from outside by the practitioner are used whatsoever. This biodynamic osteopath wrote to me because in *Stillness* I had said that biodynamic osteopaths use a subtle form of helping the potency, so I am grateful for his clarification above.

EFFERENCE ASSERTS MY WILL - NEUTRAL ARISES BY YIELDING MY WILL TO THY WILL

The practice of the neutral is to drop from the head center and orient inside our heart field while being with stillness and to sense with no agenda. Neutral also means we let all motions - inertial stuck patterns or tidal expressions - be *as it is,* which is the motion that is present. In contrast, when with efferent attention we objectify the recipient, orient to their nervous system and anatomy, name, evaluate, visualize primary respiration or any other motions, and treat symptoms, ... all of this imposes our expectations on the recipient's subtle body, which amounts to a willing-over of the recipient's already ongoing evolutionary process.

If you desire to offer post-biodynamic *Stillness Touch*, be still. That means to repose in the *presence of stillness* in non-doing; do not use efference, objectification, intention, or naming. Stop verbally negotiating hand contacts, do not create space, or establish a relational field. No orienting to the nervous system to feel cranial wave patterns, tides, midlines, and fulcra. We also refrain from trauma management, orientation to anatomy, harboring an agenda, visualizing primary respiration, or desiring a goal for the recipient, such as the relief of symptoms, or spiritual awakening. All these functional methods are appropriate when they are applied during a treatment.[18]

When our attention is efferent, we are asserting our will over the will of the recipient.

Efference places a subtle demand upon the recipient that certain events arise in them, such as Primary Respiration, health, wholeness, love, etc. Whether aware of it or not, when efferent, we are 'doing' to a client. Doing, as mentioned, confesses the egoic disposition of, "I am the intermediary between God and the recipient and I want a particular motion or state to arise in them." It is this disposition of being the doer that creates practitioner-induced false fulcra that collapse the fractal fields of the Breath of Life and Primary Respiration disappears, and is replaced by the inertial cranial wave patterns.

In a post-biodynamic practice, which means *Pure Breath of Love* is present and in charge of the session, the slightest whiff of practitioner efferent activity hinders a recipient's already ongoing evolutionary process toward wholeness. Efference also deprives a practitioner of a direct body-felt contact with the Breath of Life, even though they may long for it. It is this contradiction, and the confusion that it creates, that has motivated thousands of biodynamic graduate practitioners to enroll in our Dynamic Stillness School Initiatory, Mentor, and Post-Biodynamic courses.

Again, if you use efference, it lays down tracks of false fulcra inside you and your recipient's body. A practitioner who mistakes an empty void stillpoint for living stillness may become confused and think that the motion of the false fulcra is a part of the inherent treatment plan. When a practitioner creates an empty void that lays tracks of false fulcra inside a recipient's craniosacral system, it instills doubt about the boundless power of biodynamics. Our subtle body clearly senses this confusion.

You cannot realize neutral while objectifying a client, orienting to their nervous system, focusing on anatomy, or by mixing the three cranial methods. All of it prevents neutral from arising, which deprives you of an embodied contact with the Breath of Life. Efferent attention suffocates the potency of stillness, which shuts down the tides; what remains in the recipient are practitioner-induced false fulcra. This is why Dr. Sutherland asked practitioners to be still, meaning not to use our outer senses, do not apply any outside forces, do not test the sphenobasilar joint for lesions, all of which means a practitioner does not treat. In place of being the doer, we trust the tide and its unerring potency.

When we repose in stillness and neutral arises, the inertial motions become quiet, the cranial wave disappears, while inertial fulcra are suffused by the potency of the Breath of Life. The degree that practitioner efference subsides, determines how freely a recipient can access the wholeness emanating from the potency of the Breath of Life.

I interfere with the freedom of the recipient's inherent process of whole-making the moment I objectify, use efference, name, expect cranial wave patterns, visualize primary respiration, seek or establish midlines and fulcra, orient to the nervous system and anatomy, create space, apply conversation skills, name processes, establish a relational field, or engage in trauma management. Amid only one of these efferent practices, I limit a recipient's access to potency.[19]

Imagine if I engaged all these efferent practices during a session?

Put another way, my efferent activity is a misuse of the recipient's precious life force because efference commands that the potency of their will obeys my will. Practitioner over-willing drains the Breath of Life's potency from the recipient in the name of 'helping' them. In contrast, if I am neutral, the inertial motion naturally acquiesces to stillness, and the subsequent build-up of potency suffuses levity into the condensed inertia. The buoyancy expands the inner space of the fulcrum. When the inner space expands and becomes buoyant, the area floats to your hand and freely floats.

SENSING THE QUALITIES OF NEUTRAL INSIDE THE BODY

The presence of buoyancy is how you know the recipient's body is receiving potency.

The potency of stillness adds levity that expands space from within the fulcrum, which is the center of stillness inside the inertia. Inside this fulcrum of stillness, the potency radiates levity from the center to periphery, and the buoyancy expands and opens the inner space of the body to a suffusion of healthy fractal motion. Function optimizes, which in turn creates healthy form by shifting the shape and position of the anatomy. Amid neutral, the body self-liberates from the stress responses that assert excessive forces of gravity, which condense, compress, and constrain the freedom of fractal motion until the area expresses inertial patterns. When we abide within ourselves, poised as a fulcrum, which is a balanced point of still-ness amid the dynamic tension of opposites, we become neutral. Then, levity and gravity find harmony. The same process applies to the Breath of Life's embryological forces that make a body. The practitioner is not creating this; it is in the neutral that this process of renewal spontaneously arises.

In neutral, we sense in our inner-body atmosphere a free-floating quality that feels buoyant. This is Dr. Sutherland's hidden uncanny power that ebbs and flows amid the welling and receding potency of the entire ocean, and the seaweed freely moves with it.[20] The Breath of Life directly communicates its potent oceanic ebb and flow to the cells of the body through the ground substance, which is our inner ocean.

NEUTRAL AND ITS IMPACT ON THE GROUND SUBSTANCE

The body's ground substance is a conscious matrix - a liquid crystal medium for the intercommunication between and within all our 50 trillion cells. When an invasive force enters the body, no matter how slight, the ground substance instantly communicates its impact to every cell, which subsequently activates the nervous system's fight-flight stress response. Stress imposes an excessive force of gravity that contracts the liquid ground substance and turns it into a gel. So instead of being a free-flowing liquid crystal matrix that accurately transmits the fractal template of wholeness as the motion of health, a gelled ground substance transmits inertial motion. The resulting digital motion is holographically encoded by the limbic system, that then stores the patterns in the body's tissues, which we sense as the cranial wave. The previous transmission of the healthy fractal flow of wholeness to the cells disappears when its motions are converted to the cranial wave's digital neurological static, which adversely affects the function of all the systems in the body, which in turn disfigures the anatomy.

Instead of efference, if we orient inward, toward the heart's pacemaker near the spine it connects us to the unseen embryological forces that make the body. This radiantly awake substance of the heart field conducts the symphony of wholeness that has the power to make the body. The heart field conducts the force of health from the SA Node to the midline through the ground substance to each cell. Again, ground substance is the medium of intercommunication between the whole-making fractal motion of the Breath of Life and the 50 trillion cells of the body. When stress affects the ground substance, it informs at the speed of light every cell and organelle and the body precisely adapt to the intrusion.

Imagine how it impacts a recipient when I touch their body with an agenda.

If we harbor an agenda, realizing neutral is not possible, and the resulting inertia does not transmute to harmonious motion. Efference, orienting to the nervous system and anatomy, moving things around with the intention to shift tides in a client's body, and the use of visualization or intention at best rearranges symptoms, which will manifest other symptoms. All practitioner efferent activity shuts down the client's process of whole-making, and it depresses their immune functions. If we efferently disrupt symptoms in a client by our intention, it is a mis-using of our will, because the symptoms reappear else-where in the body. How do I know this? I successfully practiced biomechanical and functional cranial work for 20 years, and I witnessed this process.

I learned first-hand that the only way out of the trap of chasing the symptoms is to practice being neutral. That means I orient inside and quietly wait for nothing while being present in still-ness and reposed between the dynamic tension of opposites. The tension of opposites is between inertial gel and living fluid ground substance that possesses the potency to self-regulate and rebalance the body's systems when I am neutral. If I am neutral while touching, the unerring potency of stillness is transmitted to the gelled ground substance until it receives the buoyancy it needs to break free from excess gravity of inertia that compresses the fluids and creates a gel. Stillness contains the potency that adds levity, which creates space in the gelled ground substance; within the buoyancy, the inertial patterns decompress and become free to transmute the gelled ground substance back into a living fluid fractal flow.

When the contracted gel rehydrates, it becomes fluid flow that, once again, transmits the fractal information from the Breath of Life into the cells. Free-flowing fulcra transmutes inertial activity that is over-oriented to the periphery by moving the fulcra toward the center, the midline of stillness, which reconnects inertia to the stillness therein. The gelled ground substance is dis-related from the midline, and therefore, is separated from the potency of stillness. Also, contracted ground substance will distort the vertical integrity of the midline, which compromises its function of distributing life force throughout the whole body. The midline distributes the whole-making embryological forces of health from the Breath of Life to the ground substance into every cell in the body. When reposing in the dynamic tension of opposites, we are neutral amid polar activity. In neutral, we are a midline of stillness, a fulcrum.

ERICH BLECHSCHMIDT, BIODYNAMICS, AND THE WISDOM OF THE BODY

Let's talk about the midline from the perspective of conception where two polar cells, a female egg and a male sperm, unite and create a human being. Precise laws express the intelligence in the fluids as the *wisdom of the body*. We will digress here. Recall that the heart field conducts the life forces that operate in the embryonic fluids that dictate the development of the fetus, just as the heart field conducts this same information to the ground substance to maintain health in the adult body.

We have chromosomes, yet there is 'something' that is in charge beyond them that tells chromosomes to transcribe amino acid codes that create different tissues: "you become a heart," "you will be a kidney," "you are liver," "you become the left toe," and on it goes. Transcriptions occur because of the instructions from the genes. Genes are like worker bees, yet the queen bee gives them the instructions. The same principle applies in the adult: the nervous system is guided by the health in the Breath of Life.

It is obvious the nervous system did not make the body, so how can it maintain health?

Medical dogma claims that the genes make the body and that the nervous system maintains health: both notions have proven to be false.

The heart field emanates the self-existing radiance of life that conducts potency of the Breath of Life to the embryonic fluids, and it is the subsequent biodynamic activity that makes the body. The German embryologist Erich Blechschmidt (1904-1992) coined this process 'biodynamic' after he phenomenologically observed each stage of embryological development.[21] He constructed thousands of micro-thin slides of each embryonic stage from which he built 3-dimensional models of the embryo's changing shape. He observed that the metabolic activity in the fluids, the *developmental motions*, create a fetus based on many factors: the position of the cells, the type of cells that are present, how these cells touch one another, and if the touch involves compression, elongation, shear, torsion, etc. All of these factors combined create the function that makes specific anatomy to embody that function. Blechschmidt reversed the false notion that form creates function because he witnessed first-hand that it is function that creates the anatomy in the embryo. The polar forces within and between the cells possess a fluid intelligence that directs the metabolic activity in which a function occurs that in turn, creates a particular form - as anatomy - to accommodate the already existing function.

Blechschmidt calls the gestalt of wholeness *biodynamic activity*, which expresses *developmental movements* that are the energetic whirls, eddies, vibrations, and tones in the fluids that become the potent living metabolic fields of function. These metabolic fields contain the formative forces of function, which instructs the cells to become specific anatomy: the nose, a toe, face, liver, or whatever. All of these processes organize around the axial midline. The midline is a reference beam of stillness that lends the power to the functions that make the anatomy, which becomes the body. Nothing happens until there is a midline of stillness. First, there is an invisible midline, then the primitive streak appears, and the notochord grows on top of it. After the notochord grows vertically, it segments from the top down. The segments branch out and differentiate into the three primordial tissue units called mesoderm, endoderm, and ectoderm. These embryological units further differentiate to become the expressions of anatomical form, such as organs, tissues, nervous system, bones, cardiovascular, glands, lymph, ground substance, which operate as a singular, whole unit of function and form.

The first physical midline, the primitive streak, appears in the embryo between days 14 and 17. Nothing is visible in the embryo before day 14 except a clear-as-glass sphere of liquid protoplasm. Heart pacemaker cells migrate from the gut mesoderm to the periphery and surround the embryo; it is the pacemaker cells pulse that creates the motility inside the liquid embryo. It emanates vibrations from the edge of the periphery toward the center. Similar to the Taoist microcosmic orbit, as adults, the heart field emanates a holographic toroid that envelopes the body. As adults, we still have an invisible midline that is a vertical column of stillness in the center of our toroidal heart field, and we have three physical midlines: a cerebrospinal fluid-filled dural tube, a gut tube, and a notochord. These three physical midlines outwardly reflect the three invisible midlines, the *Ida*, *Pingala*, and *Sushumna* as they are known in the ancient spiritual traditions. They are negative (feminine), positive (masculine), and neutral, respectively.

After the body is formed, the notochord recedes into the center of each spinal disc and correlates with the neutral *Sushumna*. The positive pole is the cerebrospinal fluid-filled nervous system midline, which as the ascending current masculine pole correlates with *Pingala*. The negative feminine pole is *Ida*, the gut tube that emanates the descending life current that works into the embryo from the periphery to make the body. Recall that the pacemaker cells conduct this whole process by emitting the heart field's pulse that surrounds and suffuses into the embryonic protoplasm. The heart's toroid field entrains the autonomic nervous system, suffuses the neural ganglions, and concentrates them with life force. These ganglia, located in the head, throat, heart, solar plexus, abdomen, and pelvis, are known as chakra fields in spiritual traditions.

The Breath of Life emanates from the midline en masse as free-flowing fulcra; these freely moving points of stillness carry the potency, as levity, that decompress any gelled ground substance that the fulcra contact. Let's look deeper into this process. Once stillness touches the inertial motion, it becomes quiet, which liberates the fractal energy trapped in the inertia. Now the fractals free-float in a buoyant pool of fluid ground substance, which creates the healthy function that in turn restores the original anatomical form. Guess what else happens at the same time? Primary respiration reestablishes the integrity between the fluid ground substance and the midline.

When ground substance is a gel, it locally distorts or kinks the vertical shape of the midline, and when gelled ground substance liquefies, the original vertical integrity is restored to the midline, and the kinks disappear. When the midline is vertical, it is oriented to source stillness. The vertical integrity of the midline transmits the original template of healthy function to the cells of the body via the liquid ground substance. In contrast, inertial motion compromises health because the midline vertical integrity is distorted or kinked by the pull of the gelled ground substance, which adversely affects the body's functions that, in turn, distorts the anatomy. When there is vertical integrity in the midline, stillness reconnects specific areas of the body to the Breath of Life that transmits the forces of health to them. Primary respiration emanates the original blueprint template of wholeness as the fractal motions of life that create healthy function. Life force wells from the midline and recedes into the midline just like the breath does in the lungs. When fractal motion touches an inertial area of the body, it reorients to the midline, and stillness transmutes inertial motion into fractal flow. This process optimizes cellular function, which shifts the cell to an ideal position, restores its shape to accommodate the renewed healthy function. So, the Breath of Life restores healthy function that, in turn, changes the anatomical structure to accommodate it.

A SLOW-MOTION REVIEW OF THE IMPACT OF NEUTRAL

At neutral, the distorted inertial areas of the body become still. Then levity suffuses buoyancy into the inertial fulcrum that transmutes it to a free-flowing fulcrum that re-establishes healthy motion and function, which restores the ideal anatomical form. Stillness emanates potency from within the fractal motion that optimizes the functioning of the body that we are touching in neutral. If we are reposed inward, in open free attention, we can sense stillness in ourselves and in the client's whole body. Then we can sense primary respiration well and recede with a rate of 2-3 cycles per minute - as a welling of 12 seconds and 12 seconds receding that Sutherland and Becker call fluid tide.

Multidimensional welling from inside the center of stillness expands throughout the whole body. Meanwhile, potency ascends from the pelvis to the head. If your hands are on the head and sacrum as a fulcrum of stillness, during the welling and ascent, you sense the recipient's inner body space widen with potency while the space between the head and the tail draw together. During the receding and descent, the inner body narrows while the midline lengthens from head to tail. The midline breathes the Breath of Life, just like the lung breathes oxygen. During an 'in-breath,' potency ascends and shortens the midline top-to-bottom while it fattens side-to-side as the Breath of Life wells. During the descent of the Breath of Life into the body, the midline lengthens vertically and narrows side-to-side, which is why some clients will say they feel inner pressure while the potency is incarnating. If one is unaccustomed to the inner pressure of this descending current as it is embodying, it may be uncomfortable. In this case, it behooves us to bear this discomfort if we are interested in letting the Breath of Life into the body. Again, the lungs breathe air, the midline is the lung for the Breath of Life, and Dynamic Stillness is the lung of the cosmos from which breathes *Pure Breath of Love*. Keep in mind that this description is 'map.' In reality, all this happens at the same time in a paradoxical fashion that is not describable. In wholeness, there is no either-or, it is both-and, and neither at the same time. We have surveyed the neutral; now let's look at what a practitioner does to prevent *Pure Breath of Love*.

3

PRACTITIONER RECOILS THAT
IMPEDE PURE BREATH OF LOVE

D r. Carl Jung said that the subtle body of a patient is omniscient.[22] Omniscience is amplified while a recipient is suffused with *Pure Breath of Love*, so even a whiff of practitioner efferent activity during a touch session "feels intrusive, invasive, and violating." Amid efference, recipients have shared that they feel "diminished," "done to," "defiled," "violated," "manipulated." Amid efference, while in the presence of *Pure Breath of Love*, one recipient said, "My practitioner invaded my inner body space, which filled me with a painful buzzing electro-charged static."

Whenever a practitioner is efferent, orients to the nervous system, anatomy, or to the cranial wave, his awareness immediately invades the recipient's inner body. Once inside a recipient's subtle body, their heart field collapses, which, in turn, shuts down primary respiration that emanates from her heart's whole-body breathing field. As a result, the recipient is left in an empty void in which the cranial wave enters. In other words, amid a practitioner-induced collapse of the recipient's heart field, the fractal tidal expressions of primary respiration disappear. This leaves a recipient in an empty void filled with false fulcra amid the neurological static of the cranial wave.

A medical model practitioner commonly mistakes this empty void for a stillpoint, and he may misperceive that the cranial wave is the inherent treatment plan. Unfortunately, if a practitioner does not catch this error by immediately returning to neutral touch, the client's polarity may reverse, and the recipient's life current switches its direction of flow. When the life current switches directions, it shifts from a descending, grounding, embodying, and whole-making direction, to an ascending, out of the body, dissociating, separating direction. Treatment reactions can also occur, such as dizziness, nausea, headache, disorientation, lack of mental clarity, and low energy. The shift in direction of the life current also activates hypervigilance. One recipient said, "I feel trapped inside my field of hypervigilance imprisoned by anxiety."

While *Pure Breath of Love* suffuses a recipient, even the slightest practitioner efference activates the fight or flight stress response that may trigger a somatic experience of the *Core Wound*, which can re-traumatize a recipient, and create treatment reactions. [23]

Objectification, fixation of awareness on local parts, orienting to the nervous system, anatomy, or the cranial wave, these, and many other efferent activities can be the result of being trained in a medical model biodynamics for the relief of symptoms.

These practices may be appropriate when you treat a patient for symptom relief, and it may be challenging to cease efference since it is a habit. Yet, if you wish to offer Sutherland-inspired non-doing touch for the evolution of consciousness, here are some of the impediments.

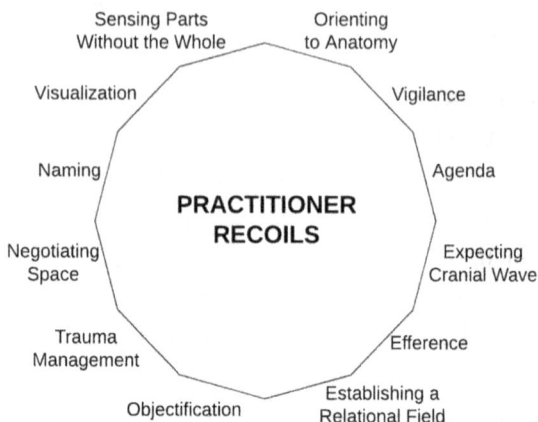

Figure 3. Specific Ways a Practitioner Recoils from Pure
Breath of Love

The following practitioner recoils impede *Pure Breath of Love*:

Orienting to Anatomy: recall that Dr. Sutherland said the unerring potency exists in the functions while Blechschmidt discovered that function makes the anatomy. In addition, Swedenborg and Russell both assert that the potency of stillness holds the blueprint template that makes the body as a whole unit. Thus, we bypass the unerring potency by attending to anatomy, which contains the *given* and is loaded with inertia. [24]

Vigilance: a practitioner may employ 'observation skills' and efferently enter into a recipient's subtle body to evaluate their nervous system or anatomy, to look for midlines, read the cranial wave motion patterns, assess the fluids, organs, or tissues, or to feel the tides. Apply any of this while inside *Pure Breath of Love*, recipients say, "it feels invasive, intrusive, and violent."

Agenda: a practitioner may harbor a treatment plan, a goal, an agenda, or use a protocol during a session. Even if well-meaning, such as you hope that the recipient gets healthier, it limits the evolutionary potential. *Pure Breath of Love* is already tenderly nudging the recipient toward wholeness in an exact tempo for their evolution. Love requires utter freedom to blossom. Here are examples of agenda:

- A practitioner wants a recipient to shift states, for example, to find neutral, or expand into the fluid tide or long tide.
- A practitioner intentionally shifts into the fluid or long tide.
- A practitioner internally suggests that a recipient enter a stillpoint.
- A practitioner orients to the nervous system or anatomy.
- A practitioner expects the cranial wave, tides, or intends techniques.
- A practitioner creates midlines, fulcra, or sends vectors into the recipient.
- A practitioner manages space (zones) or verbally negotiates contacts.
- A practitioner establishes a relational field to support a client.
- A practitioner visualizes primary respiration as the long tide that comes from the horizon "out there."

Expecting Cranial Wave: Dr. Sutherland stopped following the cranial wave once he realized the uncanny power of biodynamics. The cranial wave patterns express the nervous system's record of the past. Whereas the Breath of Life is several orders of coherence prior to the nervous system's capacities to heal. The whole-body breathing tide is steady, while the tempo of the cranial wave motion varies and is not stable. Cranial wave is a compensatory neurological impulse, and its rate shifts to reflect the functional status of the nervous system as it reacts to the stresses of life. Cranial wave motion is a local, reactive impulse that expresses the linear patterns of flexion, extension, side-bending, torsion, lateroflexion, and compression. It is not a fractal whole-body breathing tide that emanates from primary respiration.

The expectation or intending of cranial wave patterns is an efferent projection of an idea, which injects inertia into the recipient's delicate fractal field. Inertia invades their subtle body that, as false fulcra, has to be self-resolved.

When a practitioner is neutral, the cranial wave will not arise.

In contrast, when a practitioner is neutral, there are no expectations of any types of motion - even the tides or primary respiration, which leaves a client's subtle body free to express its fractal motions of life that lead to wholeness.

Objectification: is a classic medical skill. A practitioner clinically separates from the recipient and turns them into an object to treat. Objectification includes an agenda, i.e., a practitioner desires an outcome for the patient, such as the relief of symptoms, health, spiritual transformation, etc. Objectification arouses vigilance in the recipient's omniscient subtle body, which activates the nervous system's protective fight or flight defenses. When the fight or flight stress response begins, it will collapse the biodynamic breathing field of primary respiration and land the recipient in the neurological static of the cranial wave. [25]

Efference: is a subtle movement of your attention outward, under the direction of the ego and nervous system. Due to prior training, a practitioner may engage in efferent methods. Efference occurs when attention leaves your inner body space, passes through your hands, and enters the recipient's subtle body to read the status of their craniosacral system. We apply efference to orient to anatomy and the nervous system to feel the cranial wave motions in the tissues, fluids, organs, and structures of the body, or, to feel tides, midlines, stillpoints, pre-birth and birth trauma, etc. Once a practitioner trained in efference discovers cranial wave lesion patterns or any signs of trauma in the patient, he may intend cranial wave techniques - such as flexion, extension, torsion, side-bending, lateroflexion, or compression - to resolve lesions in cranial bones, dural tissues, fascia, fluids, and organs. These are classical functional cranial methods which are valuable medical treatment practices, yet they are not an aspect of a biodynamic practice according to Dr. Sutherland's definition of it.

During non-doing *Stillness Touch,* recipients report that the impact of practitioner efferent activity not only leaves them feeling "done to." They also report feeling manipulated "especially when a practitioner applies contrived motions to my body that are not happening inside me." Recipients also say that efference, "feels violating, it re-traumatized me, and created treatment reactions."

Efference is a subtle ego strategy that traps awareness in the hypermasculine disposition. If you use efference long enough, it becomes a difficult habit to break. But all is not lost if you can be still, which will naturally shift your awareness from the relief of symptoms to a non-doing practice as Dr. Sutherland taught it. Giving up efferent methods is challenging, yet by turning attention inward and being still, you can enjoy a living contact with primary respiration, which is a mandatory practice in Dr. Sutherland's biodynamics.

Naming: a practitioner may use 'conversation skills' to talk during a session by naming and describing events to the recipient as they occur. Naming disempowers a recipient and keeps them in the cranial wave. Although many recipients love conversation skills when they are in the cranial wave because it distracts them. Yet, talking prevents the necessary relaxation and inner trust required to sense and receive the subtle signals from the wisdom of their own body for guidance. Talking during a session, therefore, prevents the recipient from accessing the sufficient depth to surrender to stillness that lets *Pure Breath of Love* be in charge. Last but not least, talking during a session prevents the practitioner from realizing Dr. Sutherland's fundamental disposition: 'Be still and know.'

Establishing a Relational Field: the notion that a practitioner can negotiate a contrived relational field of empathy that supports the client contradicts the principle of being in a neutral. In neutral, a practitioner enjoys a spontaneous tonal match that is had by synchronizing with and trusting the unerring potency of the tide. When the practitioner is the doer who establishes the relational field, it is the opposite of a neutral that lets the Breath of Life be in total charge of the session. Such practitioner doing creates gross confusion about the difference between personal empathy and tonal match. Contrived empathy is achieved by the dualistic process of objectification that is generated by the practitioner's intention that creates the virtual space of a relational field. Yet it is established between a subject and object. Again, a non-doing tonal match is an attunement that occurs spontaneously by surrendering to the Breath of Life, which arises amid a practitioner neutral.

Visualization: is using intention whereby 'my will' lords over the will of the client, and subjugates the Divine Will of the Breath of Life. You cannot conceptually think, imagine, or visualize primary respiration as fluid or long tide; if you do, then what comes into existence is a virtual tide. The tides cannot and do not arise by visualizing, or by internally or externally naming them, talking about them, and you cannot shift into tide at will, except as pure fantasy inside the empty void of a virtual conceptual post-truth mind. The fluid tide wells within an enveloping field of stillness that suffuses your whole-body; this subtle fractal field is a fluid within a fluid that breathes inside and surrounds your body. When this field expands globally and becomes luminous, it is the long tide, which expresses a complex multi-dimensional luminous fractal breathing field that emanates a Radiant Presence that eventually expands and disappears into the infinity of Dynamic Stillness.

The tides are many orders of coherence beyond nervous systems' capacity. You sense tides only with heart perception by synchronized entrainment.

Negotiating Space: a practitioner negotiates the space between themselves and the recipient. The practitioner imagines zones of space that supposedly correlate with a specific tidal field in the name of supporting the recipient's sense of safety and containment. For example, a practitioner contrives an expanded space of the long tide by visualizing it. However as mentioned, it is impossible to intend, negotiate, or visualize a living, tonally matched space or a tidal zone even for yourself, much less for a recipient you barely know. You cannot negotiate tides or visualize them; they arise inherently within their respective zones of stillness when we yield to neutral.

To repeat: the tidal fields are orders of coherence beyond the capacities of your brain. By grace, you sense tides in neutral by heart perception.

A practitioner's neutral touch is crucial while the fluid flow transitions into the vast luminosity, which is a transpersonal realm of consciousness. Hence, anytime a practitioner intentionally negotiates a space by visualizing a tidal zone, it impinges on a recipient's omniscient subtle body and they will feel objectified by the practitioners' efference. *Stillness Touch* recipients report sensing invasiveness when the practitioner's attention enters their personal sacred inner body space. Recall that Dr. Carl Jung said the recipient's subtle body is omniscient under normal therapeutic circumstances; imagine the degree of omniscience in the presence of *Pure Breath of Love*: the subtle body is infinitely more sensitive, exquisitely delicate, refined, and vulnerable. Many recipients report that when a practitioner efferently creates a negotiated space it "feels smothering, restrictive, compressive, contrived, violent, and manipulative because it does not match my space that I am in." Negotiating space repels *Pure Breath of Love*.

Trauma Management: trauma management is an excellent medical method that works with nervous system mechanisms that organize trauma. Some practitioners manage various traumas in a recipient, be it pre-birth, birth, or post-birth trauma by using various techniques such as breathing, dialogue, movement, and visualizations to cultivate the sense of safety and grounding in the client. Given that the practice of trauma management is a medical method it has no place in a non-doing biodynamic practice. It is the Breath of Life that minimizes the effects of trauma the moment it occurs, so it can unravel all trauma in a recipient without our help if we touch in neutral.

Following Parts Without Sensing the Whole: warning - we will be using biodynamic terminology. Let's suppose you are not orienting to the nervous system or anatomy, nor are you being guided by the cranial wave, and you are not intending cranial wave techniques for the relief of symptoms. Instead, you orient to the stillness within, connect with the *fluid tide*, and are following its *fluid drive* while appreciating the *motion present*. However, there is a caveat: if your awareness is not also simultaneously synchronized with the whole-body field of *primary respiration*, you fall into the trap of unconsciously creating inertial motions that leave *false fulcra* in the client - even if you are engaged in a biodynamic session.

In other words, if most of your awareness is NOT synchronized with the global potency that wells inside and beyond your whole-body breathing field as *primary respiration*, and you are only focusing on the local activities inside the recipient, then you are tracking inertial motion. What? Yep, even during an authentic biodynamic session, if you are following the fluids it does not reveal the living potency of the tides or its inherent evolutionary plan. Recall that *potency* is a global presence that expresses the forces of life, health, and wholeness in both the practitioner and the recipient. *Potency*, again, is a subtle substance, a living *fluid within a fluid*, as Sutherland characterizes it. Unless potency is in total charge of a session, we get caught in the trap of being the doer who wants to know what the Breath of Life is up to, which is not our business. A more subtle trap occurs when a practitioner attempts to intuit what the Breath of Life is about to do next; although it seems like we are leaving the Breath of Life in charge, by our anticipation, we become the doer and get in the way. As Dr. Becker said, "When you are dealing with the highest known energy that's available, it does not want anyone interfering with what it is trying to do."[26]

The art to sensing potency is orient inside, be still, wait for nothing, amid don't know. If you orient inside and wait for nothing, your attention will repose in a soft, unfocused, unfixed, free, open awareness. Then, by grace, the invisible potency of the Breath of Life gently swaddles your attention and reveals herself to you. Her motions move your attention, which becomes your inner-body guide during a session. Your free attention moves with the potency of the Breath of Life as it expresses as primary respiration from the midline and distributes its fractal motion to the whole-body, suffusing coherent, healthy function to all systems in you, and the recipient's entire bodily being.

When sensing *primary respiration* inside yourself as it arises, it feels like a subtle breathing of your consciousness, while potent life force wells up and down the midline. At the same time, life force expands and recedes throughout the whole body in all directions simultaneously.

> When your attention synchronizes and moves with primary respiration, the subsequent potency moves your hands from place to place on the recipient, but you are not doing it.

In summary, although *fluid tide primary respiration* contains the *fluid drive*, it is distinct from it. *Fluid drive* moves like a flowing river within the ocean of *primary respiration*. *Primary respiration* is a global whole-body field of *potency* that invisibly shifts the local *fluid drive* from *fulcrum*-to-*fulcrum* inside the client's subtle inner-body breathing field. When the *potency* inside the *fluid drive* dwells in a particular local fulcrum in the recipient to resolve inertia, that activity is called the *motion present*, which will inherently resolve specific inertial motions in those areas, which positively affect the whole body. The practitioner is doing nothing except repose in the *presence of stillness* within, while the Breath of Life engages its process of *transmutation*.

In contrast, inertial motions of the cranial wave automatically repeat digital patterns that, like photographs, are frozen in time. Inertia maintains itself by draining the *potency* of the life forces from the body. In contrast, the *potency* of *primary respiration transmutes* lifeless inertial digital patterns, restoring them to their original free-flowing fractal state. Places in the body where there is inertia turns the liquid ground substance into a gel state, which emits digital motion. However, potency transmutes gelled ground substance back into a liquid and the digital inertial patterns of the cranial wave emitted by gel transmute by dissolving into living fractals.

Living potency transmutes ground substance from a gel to fluid. Liquid ground substance accurately transmits the fractal information that conveys to the cells the template of wholeness that emanates from the potency of the Breath of Life.

One of Sutherland's famous analogies, the *Tour of the Minnow*, points to the Breath of Life's indescribable process of transmutation in the nervous system.[27] If we expand his tour to a biodynamic perspective, the specific path of the fish in a pond as it moves from place to place is the fluid drive. The fish's particular undulating body motility in a specific location in the pond where it dwells is the motion present, and the entire motion of the pond is primary respiration. If you only focus on the journey of the fish in the pond, the fluid drive, or on its specific bodily gestures, the motion present, as interesting as it may be, without the larger perspective that includes awareness of the effects of the global motion of the entire pond as the forces of potency, you lose the perspective of wholeness. Potency reveals the whole Gestalt of the inherent treatment plan, i.e., why the fish is moving where it does in the pond to dwell in a specific location. To appreciate the Breath of Life's inherent treatment plan:

> Let all three aspects simultaneously dwell in your awareness - Primary Respiration, fluid drive, motion present - in neutral, amid a repose in non-doing and not knowing.

We are sincere practitioners, and we long to help the Breath of Life heal the fish, so we are tempted to nudge the fish a bit, and direct it along its path because we want to fix the bodily lesion patterns that cause it suffering. We train and we have treatment skills: we know how to orient to the nervous system, to the anatomy, and to cranial wave patterns to relieve symptoms. Fair enough, that is functional cranial work, a great service; but if we want to practice a non-medical approach that evolves consciousness, we need to have the discipline and courage to be still and wait for nothing, in unknowing.

Then we enter what Dr. Jealous calls the mysterious metabolic fields of life, which move in a perpetual fractal flow, guided by primary respiration. These fractal motions express the original template of wholeness that bestows health moment by moment, and they are not predictable. This motion of life possesses the ancient cumulative cellular consciousness that is inherent to all living organisms. Indeed, I hope you can agree that Primordial Intelligence is capable of resolving the dilemma of the fish without our generous, yet misguided, assistance?

> Functional cranial work is a beautiful practice, but do not call it biodynamic. Telling a client that you offer biodynamic when it is not is unethical conduct.

As practitioners, if we trained to help out the Breath of Life, we are innocent. However, we must give that up to practice non-doing biodynamic cranial for the evolution of consciousness the way that Dr. Sutherland taught.

You have to give up all the efferent methods that you learned in your cranial training. Again Dr. Becker: "When you are dealing with the highest known energy that's available, it does not want anyone interfering with what it is trying to do."

Once Dr. Sutherland realized how "uncanny" the potency and the power of a non-doing practice was, he altogether ceased orienting to the nervous system and to its cranial wave expressions. He stopped using intention to direct the tides to correct lesion patterns, to treat, and relieve symptoms. His uncanny experiences showed Sutherland how the potency of the tides heal without a practitioner adding anything.

Repeated contact with the potency of the Breath of Life leads to the realization of Dynamic Stillness, which, like a second birth, delivers you into an inner beyond that unites your body and consciousness with *Pure Breath of Love.*

Even if we refrain from engaging the practices that recoil the *Pure Breath of Love,* and we can access neutral, how do we know we are in a biodynamic session?

Let's explore some of the ways to verify if we are in the biodynamic domain.

QUALITIES OF A BIODYNAMIC SESSION
(BIODYNAMIC TERMS ARE IN ITALICS)

- A biodynamic session begins when you sense a field of stillness envelope and suffuse your whole inner body space, while *primary respiration* emanates a subtle breath from within the stillness.
- *Fluid* and *long tide* express inner breath within a corollary matching field of stillness. Each tidal expression ebbs and flows in a precise breathing tempo, inside a specific enveloping field of stillness that correlates with a particular state of consciousness.
- Stillness emanates from the midline into the inner body space, then it expands globally to infinity. Beyond infinity, your consciousness implodes while *Dynamic Stillness* suffuses your cells with consciousness and you realize the Consciousness of the Whole that contains all enfoldments of consciousness.
- When your awareness expands infinitely inside the body, you realize infinitesimal stillness in each cell.

Meanwhile, your body also expresses infinite consciousness.

- Paradoxical Consciousness occurs when the parts and whole are simultaneous and inclusive; this is known as both/and.
- You sense consciousness in earth, water, air, fire, ether, that combine to become a quintessential element of consciousness as Pure Breath of Love.
- Repeated contact with the *fluid tide* lifts awareness freeing it from the trap of the narcissistic ego; then contact with the *long tide* expands awareness into a global witness consciousness. Perception shifts from witnessing to being witnessed by the Self, and then the Self, I AM becomes your perception. I AM then unites with Primordial Mother Love that creates all that is. You realize an inner union between Body, Pure Consciousness, and the tender Mother Love.
- Beyond the imploded inner-body infinity of *Dynamic Stillness*, post-biodynamics begins with the realization of Pure Breath of Love, which dissolves all *tides* and enfoldments of consciousness, and combines them into a single alchemical super substance that suffuses your cells, renews your consciousness, and unites your body and consciousness with all that is. Since the *fluid* and *long tides* are no longer perceived, Stillness Touch is a post-biodynamic practice.
- The inclusiveness of your consciousness in post-biodynamics is beyond words, mapless, nameless, and paradoxical - a state of both/and, and neither all at once.
- Your realizations in Pure Breath of Love are paradoxical. For example, all at the same time you can realize union with all your aspects, with nature, and the elements while you are in contact with extraordinary transpersonal sensory, visual, audio, gustatory,

olfactory, and tactile qualities that combine as one, and your whole body becomes an organ of perception. This is known as Spiritual Touch by which you are connected with The All. Here you can be present to any degree of intensity, intimacy, and paradox while you face, unite with, and integrate all aspects of your Core Erotic Wound. [28]

- A daily *Stillness Practice* gradually leads to the realization of *Pure Breath of Love*, and now we can explore some of the practices below.

4

STILLNESS PRACTICES

The next two chapters explore *Stillness Practices* that are based on the ancient spiritual practice called *Pratya-hara*. Millions of people have meditated this way daily for billions of hours over thousands of years. *Pratyahara* is orienting your awareness inward to contact the Divinity within that inherently connects with the outer Divine. The benefit of this daily regular meditative practice is that consciousness grad-ually exhibits the subtle *inner breaths* of your self-existing heart radiance. In time, your heart radiance connects with your pelvic center that expresses the sensuous *Eros* that wells from the hidden depths of the Divine Feminine power, which is known as the *Kundalini*, or the *Sacred Force of Love*. When the heart and pelvic essences unite, it ignites an alchemical substance of consciousness that is one with love. Tantric Buddhists call this substance the *innate bliss*. *Innate bliss* is also known as *prajna*, the wisdom of the body, that in Christianity is the *Sophia*, while in depth psychology it is *Eros*.

Innate bliss is a highly refined alchemical substance of consciousness that suffuses your subtle body with an illuminative *inner breath.* Its potent presence frees charged emotions that are trapped as subtle body knots, which distribute patterns of armor in the flesh. The patterns of armor distributed in the body provides a map of how your consciousness has fragmented into pieces, and how each piece displays unsavory defensive behaviors that recoil consciousness from love. Once *innate bliss* suffuses the inner body, it melts the subtle body knots, softens the body armor, transmutes gelled ground substance to a liquid, and the *Sacred Power of Love* awakens in your cells.

The fragmented aspects of consciousness also display symptoms of an inner war between your three primary body centers of head, heart, and pelvis. Innate bliss illuminates the strategies in each of these centers, which collectively recoil your body-felt awareness away from love. You can evolve beyond the conditioned limits that these conflicts impose on you by being present to them. At the same time, you can face and be with your shadows while innate bliss illuminates and liberates the inertial patterns that fragment consciousness.

Each aspect of the shadow that we face and integrate contributes to our wholeness. First the shadow becomes a gift that then deepens into our unique powers, the Siddhis.

TRANSMUTE YOUR SHADOW - DISSOLVE THE INNER WAR

When the three primary body centers head, heart, and pelvis are at war, it creates an inner battle between thinking, feeling, and will, which fragments consciousness.

> *In the head, the shadow is* doubt.
> *In the heart, the shadow is* hatred.

The shadow in the pelvis is fear,
which paralyzes your will.

If you wish to restore your consciousness to wholeness, it is essential that you navigate all aspects of your shadow by practicing *Pratyahara*. Every day you sit, repose inward, and wait, until eventually you sense *innate bliss* with the whole of your attention. *Innate bliss* illuminates all aspects of your shadow. You face your shadow by merely being present to its uncomfortable manifestations of intensity. Gradually, by being present, the inner war ends, and your sense of separation dissolves, which ends ego's control over your body's three primary centers that fragmented your consciousness. However, as a reminder, to enjoy the fruits of this unified consciousness requires that you engage a regular, daily sitting practice. Also, as we will address later, there is a deeper shadow to face that creates the core aspects of your personality that *unconsciously* recoil you from love. This shadow comes from the *Core Erotic Wound*, also known as the *Grail Wound*. It is essential to thoroughly navigate your core wound if you desire to become a whole spectral human-being.[29]

LOVE IS THE UNRESTRICTED FLOW OF LIFE FORCE IN THE BODY

Eventually, after the practice of *Pratyahara* bears fruit, you acclimate to the power of love pulsing in your body - *if you do not project your desire onto an object* for self gratification, love implodes into the cells and you enjoy an erotic unity with the All.

When Eros freely flows, the body, consciousness, and love reunite.

WHAT HINDERS AN UTTER BODILY UNION WITH CONSCIOUSNESS AND LOVE?

Union is hindered by the recoils, which are unconscious blocks in the body and psyche that restrict the free-flow of *Eros*. But these blocks are not the cause; they are effects of the *Core Erotic Wound* as well as the subsequent inner conflicts between the three primary bodily centers of head, heart, pelvis.

Again, these blocks arise due to a war-like reactivity that rages inside the three centers between the masculine and feminine principles - *pingala* and *ida* - that when in harmony are polar expressions of the *Sacred Force of Love*, the *Kundalini*. However, when these poles conflict, it blocks the free-flowing pulse of love, which is the source of our suffering.

Hermes' Caduceus symbolizes this motif. Two snakes, the masculine - *pingala* and the feminine - *ida* intertwine and wrap around a midline column of stillness - the *Sushumna*. The two snakes cross each of the seven chakras that together emanate our full spectral, spiritual-psycho-emotional-physical nature. When there are conflicts between *ida* and *pingala* they display the shadow elements that are hidden within each chakra region that adversely affect our wholeness: we suffer narcissistic thoughts, feelings, and emotions, foggy cognition, decreased immunity, tight fascia, armor in the muscles and organs that restrict the flow of blood, lymph, cerebrospinal fluid, and the fluid ground substance becomes a gel, etc.. All this creates imbalances in the meridians, bindu points, and the midline. The inner war is also expressed in the three primary centers of head, heart and pelvis that respectively express *doubt*, *hatred*, and *fear*, which activate the shadows hidden in each chakra. Add the psycho-somatic recoils from love due the *Core Erotic Wound*, and the practitioner recoils that impede *Pure Breath of Love* and you can see we have a lot to face.[30]

But how do we face all this? With presence.

Amid a surrender to what is, if with *presence* you can be with the uncomfortable aspects of your shadow while orienting inward daily, it decreases the paralyzing power that the shadow has on your will that leaves you afraid to act. Gradually, all aspects of your shadow transmute into its original essence as your gifts. However, it is challenging to recognize, face, and *feel* the discomfort while all the unsavory aspects of your shadow undergo transmutation.

> *As a ferocious act of the will, utterly surrender your body to love, which occurs if you let love have all of you as a sacred offering, amid the expressions of your shadow.*

A MEDITATIVE CHALLENGE

One challenge during your regular daily meditation practice of *Pratyahara,* occurs when inner buoyancy arises and expands consciousness in your inner body space.

Once the expansion of your consciousness surpasses the boundaries of your known inside infinite stillness, the head, heart, and pelvis centers split apart and fly in all directions. This event is extremely chaotic, disorienting, and intensely uncomfortable; yet, it is necessary to bear with presence because it loosens the powerful grip that ego has over your three centers. Your task is to remain inwardly present, grounded, and centered while you bear the intensity of this whole-making, disintegration-reintegration process. When the three centers reunite, their original essential powers are renewed and can freely be expressed. In other words, by facing your shadow you restore your power.

After you reintegrate the renewal of your three centers, your presence-of-will becomes so strong that you can remain inwardly anchored in your body while the *innate bliss* softly melts the shadow material held in the body as armor. When the body armor dissolves, it releases the stored emotional aspects of the shadow, and the trapped *Eros* is liberated, which then softens the subtle body knots that recoil your awareness from love. Once the subtle body's knots of recoil melt, the central channel opens, and its potency liberates the remaining blocked areas. An open central channel strengthens the potency of your radiant heart consciousness while your body is being suffused by the vibrant silence of love. When all three centers re-unite, it restores our original inner harmony and wholeness.

So, facing your shadow is essential for self-realization. Yet, as you can see, it is not for the faint of heart. To transmute ego's narcissistic grip on your awareness, you not only remain inwardly present to be with intensity, chaos, disorientation, intimacy, and paradox while your shadow is being illuminated; you also bear the discomfort of *knowing thyself* while *innate bliss* illuminates the details of how you acted out your shadow aspects in the past.

> *No wonder ego avoids the Completion Stage at all costs. Ego is unable to be with the intensity of emotions so it uses doubt, hatred, and fear to stop the evolutionary process because self-knowledge is too horrifying to bear.*

CONFRONTING EGO'S STRATEGIES OF RECOIL FROM LOVE

Again, one of your most difficult challenges is to confront the ego's strategies that recoil your awareness from love. Most strategies are unconscious, and hidden in the soma, so it is up to the unwavering quality of your presence to catch the grasping and avoidance strategies of the mind along with the ego's subtle control games that create your limiting personality quirks.

More challenging is to face and feel the secret drives and needs of the shadow that recoil you away from intimate love and relatedness.

Again, all of these combined aspects of the shadow arise from the disharmony in the subtle body chakra fields, which creates the powerful psychological complexes that possess profound intensity. It is the power of the intensity that hinders you from summoning the strength of will to remain *present*. It is *presence* that frees your awareness from the narcissistic grip of ego that, when liberated, allows you to cross the threshold and *know thyself* in the full spectral glory of wholeness.

When you are receptive to and can *sense* the unsavory aspects of your shadow, while each aspect is being illuminated by *innate bliss*, you may experience intense doubt, hatred, terror, and rage. The degree of intensity is so shocking that you think, "This can't be me." Yet your full spectrum nature *includes* the deepest, most dreaded shadow *and* your unbearable radiantly awake *Self*. If you can bear the intensity of *knowing thyself*, then *all* your aspects unite with universal love and connect you with all of creation.

One pitfall on the journey to love is the by-pass that occurs due to the lack of willpower. When the will collapses, awareness dissociates, and the ego seeks refuge in the 'non-dual' disposition that declares, "I am not my body." In contrast, an embodied realization knows your body to be love's most exquisite creative expression. You realize *Criatura* when your heart's mysterious inner space emanates its self-existing radiance that is connected to *Eros* in your pelvis that unites body, consciousness, and love.[31]

> When Shiva and Shakti unite as formless and form, your touch transmits love to others.

CRIATURA IS WHOLENESS OF THE BODY IN EROTIC UNITY WITH THE ALL

Amid a spectral realization of *Criatura,* offering *Stillness Touch* for the evolution of consciousness transmits universal love to a recipient. A recipient can see through the ego's false notion that the body is made of discrete material anatomical parts that are separate from consciousness (*Shiva*) and love (*Shakti*). Separation does not exist in a spectral body. As noted, being separate is a misperception of the ego, which breaks wholeness into parts, which recoil you from love. As mentioned, recoil occurs because the ego is terrified of contacting the bewildering intensity of the power of the Divine Feminine that creates the spectral union between body, consciousness, and love.

> *Love is invisible flesh that becomes visible as the body. Abide inwardly in stillness to be with your sensations, and realize that the body is an expression of boundless love.*

Stillness Touch is a path of development for realizing that body-is-love. Whether you sit in stillness daily, or you give and receive *Stillness Touch* sessions, the challenge is to remain present inwardly to sense the profound intensity that arises while you repose inwardly in stillness. Attend to the sensations in your inner body space - its rhythms and qualities - without internally naming, understanding, transforming, expecting, or doing anything with them.

> Whatever arises inside you, *let it be* and *let it in.*

Attend to the sensations that ebb and flow inside your body until your attention is free from fixation, recoil, and over-enamor. Then your attention is neutral, and it is free to move with the *inner breaths* of your heart's self-existing radiance that suffuses the body with love. With freed attention, you can effortlessly be with all the ways your body expresses its infinite spectral nature. The body in its spectral wholeness is inclusive of everything: the ascending and descending life currents, the zones of emotional tension, body armor, intensity, intimacy, paradox, thoughts, feelings, memories, shock, spaciousness, fluidity, luminosity, emptiness, spiritual states, erotic sensuousness, tones, the core wound, Dynamic Stillness, *Eros*, the *Sacred Tremor, Pure Breath of Love*, again, nothing is excluded.

Presence awakens your heart perception: when your hearts' subtle *inner breaths* well and recede, they caress, soften, and transmute everything your presence attends to. Your presence breathes the living fractals of your heart's self-existing radiance, which is the Divine Feminine Wisdom that when she unfolds throughout you, you realize non-separate consciousness. This is opposite to the ego's hypermasculine strategies of separation that objectify, break wholeness into parts, and use efference to intend, control, name, and manipulate what is present due to the terror of the whole-making force of love.[32]

TOUCH AS TRANSMISSION

Inner body tones emanate from *within* your heart field to transmit the power of love. The transmission of an embodied consciousness that is non-separate from love occurs wordlessly, beyond thinking, knowing, naming, or understanding.

> *Transmission is because the infinite coherence of your heart field invokes the laws of entrainment. The medium for entrainment is a neutral touch that transmits an invisible substance that co-breathes love flesh-to-flesh from one body to the other.*

You develop receptivity to this invisible substance of unifying potency by your daily practice of *Pratyahara* as a reversing of your efference. Again, efference is the habitual outward flow of your attention that is directed to the nervous system and anatomy while touching another. To reverse efference, orient inwardly and sense the qualities of stillness in the atmosphere of your inner body space. Then repose in an open-hearted receptivity to the transmission that's already active inside your inner body field.

More specifically, orient your attention inward toward the back of the heart at the pacemaker, or sinoatrial node (SA node) near the spine: this is your center, the fulcrum that reawakens your whole body as a sensing organ of perception. After you acclimate to the surging power of your heart radiance, you add an advanced practice of effortlessly reposing in the sensuousness of *Eros* in your pelvic floor. If you repose in the *Eros* that wells from your pelvis while you connect with your heart radiance without letting the recoils of doubt, hatred, or fear move you away from *Eros*, then your inner body space will expand with love inside. Within your expanded inner body space of love, Dynamic Stillness will implode, and the bottom drops out of your pelvis, creating an inner body infinity in which *Pure Breath of Love* descends into and suffuses all of your cells.

> In Pure Breath of Love, the recipient and practitioner are not separate; so, your guidance to where to touch, its quality, and for how long is flawless.

THE HEART IS THE FULCRUM, THE CENTER OF THE SELF

Repose, and soak up the qualities in your heart field, let them impact you, which connects you to infinite potency. After repeated contact with your hearts' radiant potency, you realize that the qualities in the atmosphere *inside* your heart field are the same as the qualities outside. To land in this embodied realization, allow your awareness to sink from your head and repose in your heart field while you sense the qualities, or tones, in your *inner body*. Be receptive to and absorb all the qualities that you sense in the space of your inner body. In other words, *let it in*, and allow the tonal qualities in your inner body atmosphere to touch and impact you without internally naming, thinking about, trying to understand, going after, changing, or resisting them:

Just be with what is, as it is, while you let it into your inner body.

STILLNESS PRACTICE: REPOSE IN THE DYNAMIC TENSION OF OPPOSITES

Holding awareness steady between the polarities of levity and gravity bring you to a natural state of balance, the neutral. Objectification, over enamor, fear, recoil, doubt, hatred, or an adversarial disposition toward either the masculine, feminine, or neutral pole creates separation, which is dualistic and one-sided. Dualism fragments your consciousness into parts and destabilizes it, which prevents you from enjoying the full capacities of unwavering presence that can effortlessly *be with what is*.

Unwavering presence keeps you in constant contact with your original indestructible innocence. The word unwavering can be misleading if it is taken to mean unmoving, rather than as the capacity to stay present amid all change.

Indestructible Innocence is the capacity to *be with what is as it is* regardless of its intensity. As an expressed aspect of love, you can be *present* amid any intensity without distancing, objectification, over enamor, recoil, shut down, dissociation, projection, transference, countertransference, or trying to understand, name, manipulate, visualize, change either the situation, yourself, or others to feel safe. You cultivate an ever-increasing capacity to be present while the body unites with love as an unbroken continuity of consciousness regardless of what is happening.

This life-long practice is not a goal you reach.

Again, cultivating an unwavering presence means to *be with what is - as it is -* which is the practice that strengthens your will. You can then behold in unconditional regard any degree of intensity, intimacy, or paradox that manifests while you receive and offer *Stillness Touch.* Unwavering presence is available when you sit in meditation alone, you are in a group field, in the marketplace, the household, and when you give or receive intimate touch. The practice of touch possesses greater intensity, which further strengthens your unwavering presence. Once you can repose inwardly amid intimacy, it is a portal to love.

To repeat, an unwavering presence grants you the ability to *feel* the intensity and *be with it, as it is,* which is a path to intimacy with self, with another, in life, and with love. As your capacity to *be with - as it is -* stabilizes, it becomes a permanent faculty of your heart perception. Gradually, an unwavering presence becomes *Indestructible Innocence,* a capacity to be with *what is* while remaining in constant contact with love with an undefended heart that is enveloped in reverence and awe.

As noted in the book *Stillness,* heart perception becomes a transparent eye, an illuminative faculty by which you see the spiritual *through the body.*[33] You realize that the body itself is an organ of perception that is in *Spiritual Touch* with everything. In this disposition, you are not afraid to bear the dark and tragic aspects of your shadow, others' shadow, or the horrifying aspects of human existence; regardless of life's intensity, your inner body contact with love remains constant.

You naturally cultivate the precise discernment to choose what nurtures your heart's body-felt sense, and you have the strength of will to avoid what erodes it. As your choices orient toward the cultivation of heart perception, your unwavering presence stabilizes, and your body realizes its transpersonal power that is a sacred sense known as *Spiritual Touch* that unites you with The All. You then enjoy a conscious, unbroken, embodied contact with all of life's flow of love, which moves you.

You feel suspended in a *boundless sea of love* that is your inexhaustible wellspring of creativity, which bubbles behind consciousness as its source that pervades all things and erotically expresses as the flesh of your body.

Stillness Practices by being with levity and gravity, the opposites unite.

Levity Practices	Neutral	Gravity Practices
Head Stillness	Heart Stillness	Repose in the Pelvis
Whole-Body Breathing	Midline Meditation	Repose in Feelings and Emotions

A BODY AS CONSCIOUSNESS MEDITATION

The first recommendation is to sit every day for some time (suggested is 45 minutes) practicing *Pratyahara*. That means you orient attention inside and down, below the neck somewhere inside the body space, and sense whatever arises - even if nothing arises, continue to sense it. If *Pratyahara* is without agenda, is sincere, and without recoil due to ego tricks, then eventually your presence unites with the power that is prior to the body, which is the Divine Feminine Will that created all things. In the Vedas, this living inner presence is considered to be the Divine Will. In the Christian faith, it is the *Sophia*, the Holy Wisdom of the World, and in Buddhism it is the *Prajna-paramita*, while Taoism calls it *Shen*. The Divine Feminine is also the same mysterious embryonic force that makes the body. If we contact the Feminine Wisdom within us, she guides our will and takes charge of our body, speech, and mind.

After our *Stillness Practice* fructifies, and our inner contact with the Divine Feminine is consistent, then when we can engage the 5-minute preparatory practice that lets the Divine Will lead the session during *Stillness Touch*. Our mini-preparation deeply impacts the person lying down. So just before touching someone, we prepare, which can be done sitting or standing as a mini-version of our daily 45-minute sitting practice. Once our presence inwardly contacts the mysterious power that is prior-to-body, one begins touching based on the guidance from movements of the inner breaths. One refrains from being guided by the nervous system, anatomy, or by unconscious recoil from the ego's hidden needs to avoid contact with the subtle Breaths. We need to develop a daily meditation routine before we can engage our mini-practice. Below is one sugges-tion on how to sit daily; however, you will find your own way of navigating the order of your inner meditative process that works best for you.

A DAILY PRACTICE

Here is one way to practice meditation: Sit straight yet relaxed in a way that allows your flesh to soften and sink inward toward your inner body space, while letting your inner-body buoyancy swaddle your body. Let your sense gates - sight, hearing, smell, taste, touch - become receptive by orienting them inward. Your sense gate inner receptivity will spread into your whole inner body space, and the whole body will become an inner sensing organ of perception. Withdraw the nervous system's radar-like outer flow of your attention; let your awareness recede inside your brain core. Relax the nervous system's vigilance, and soften ego's need to know if the environment is safe. Instead, *repose in an openhearted relaxation* as you attend *inwardly* and *sense* the *darkness of matter* inside your body.

PERINEUM INNER BREATHING PORTAL

Let all the above continue on its own, during your *whole-body breathing*. To practice whole-body breathing, gather your *sensing* awareness into a small point in the center of the *inner space* of your perineum. During each in-breath within the point, *sense* how the space expands, like filling a balloon from *inside to out*, from the center to periphery. Do not visualize this, *sense* it happening from within the point in which you are breathing inside. On each out-breath, *inhabit* the expanded *space* inside the point that is created by the in-breath, and sense the qualities here. Let your attention repose in this newly expanded point in your inner-body pelvic space. Do this until *inner breath fills the space in your body*. Feel this with your sensing presence. It might take several minutes for this to occur.

> Instead of you doing the breathing, you may feel that you are being breathed. Relax and let it be *as it is*.

Let the whole-body inner breathing in the perineum continue by itself. At the same time, place your attention at the crown of your head: open the crown and *receive* infinite stillness and let it cascade into your brain, like a gentle waterfall. As your breathing *presence of stillness* descends, let your brain surrender its vigilance until it becomes *receptive* and soaks up like a sponge the tonal qualities of stillness without internally naming any of the qualities. Remain mindful that the whole-body inner breathing in the pelvis is on-going while you attend to the brain and spinal cord as one unit that is absorbing the stillness as your sensing awareness cascades down. After a while, let your *sensing* awareness land in your heart space. Continue to *sensually receive* all the tonal qualities that are present in the atmosphere of your entire inner body space from your inner breathing in the head and pelvis.

In the heart, move your *sensing* awareness toward the back of the heart near the spine, and at the same time, continue to *sense the atmosphere in your entire inner body space*. Your *inner breath* micro-senses as an inner navigation at the heart's pacemaker, the SA Node at the spine. You do not look for or visualize this area; you *sense* with your inner breath near the spine without expectation.

When inner sensing is slow enough, you can savor the subtle nuances of sensation *within* your heart near the spine, and you may sense a breathing *presence* arising from a tiny invisible inner breathing portal. You sense this invisible substance as a subtle *breathing* into your inner body space that passes to-and-fro through the tiny portal at the back of the heart. This *prana breath* fills your entire inner body space with a buoyancy-suffused tender, sensuous flow.

> You learn effortless *sensing concentration* that you strengthen by a daily repetition of your heart field navigation.

When reposing *at the back of the heart* with your *sensing* awareness, the "I" or Soul, attends *inwardly* to the delicate activity of the *inner heart field,* which breathes the primordial substance of life, as *prima materia* or *prana,* from your inner heart space that fills your whole body.

Here, while reposing *in the heart field*, you *sensually* attend to the micro-nuanced qualities that feel like tones in your *inner body space*. Do not inwardly name or try to make meaning out of these tonal micro-qualities, nor do you attend to your thoughts, the issues of your Soul, emotions, or even sleep. If you can *let it all be*, then everything will pass like clouds in the sky, without the ego needing to grasp or avoid the qualities that are here. *Receive* the impact of the sensual qualities of tenderness that breathe through your opened-heart space.

> Do not stop your thoughts, emotions, or other activities, nor attend to them. Let it be, leave it as it is, let go into open hearted repose amid 'don't know.'

While *sensually* abiding in the inner breathing portal at the back of the heart, you may become aware of various expressions *inside* the space of your body that affects your flesh. It can be pain, stiffness, tightness, areas of dis-ease, oscillations of different kinds of fast and short rhythmic pulsations, vibrations, electrostatic charge, the heartbeat, and breath rhythms, thoughts, feelings, emotions, memories, worries, and other revelations of the body. These are expressions of the neurological impulse, the cranial wave, that displays the sympathetic nervous system's reactivity to the stress and anxiety that is stored in your tissues.

> The practice is to hang out, and sensually be inside and with all this activity *as it is*. If awareness recoils, and rises into the head, let it sink and re-orient your attention to the back of the heart.

The most challenging part of this self-practice, initially, is learning to hang out in the *inner body space* to sense these qualities long enough amid the intensity, and not recoil into the head and start thinking or trying to figure it out. Otherwise, you may get lost in thinking, grasping, enamor, avoidance, naming, talking, visualizing, fantasy, recoil, rapid bodily movements, ego control, dissociation, desire, emotionality, or you may go to sleep. Regardless of what's here, repose, *let it all be*, and *leave it as it is*.

In time, the relationship between your sensing presence and the intensity of the tissues' neurological activity begins to bear fruit, and the motion will transmute from a digital, static-like electrical quality to a sensuous inner body flow, while your consciousness expands and unfolds *as* an expression of the body.

While resting at the back of the heart near the spine, your sensing awareness rides to-and-fro on the whole-body *inner breath*, while you attend to the inner body's sensuous rhythmic expressions. Continue to inwardly orient attention toward the inner breathing portal at the back of your heart. Gradually there will be a *presence*, a *strong sense* of 'I' that is oriented inwardly, which abides in the back of the heart and attends to the sensuous awareness of your inner body qualities.

INNER-BODY FLOW

At some point, you realize that the relationship between your awareness and the sensuous inner body flow is like a wordless conversation, or a negotiation between a vigilant rapid nervous system tissue motion and a much slower relaxed, sensuous fluid whole-body motion of the inner body prana. You may be aware that the elegant fluid flow has a bittersweet quality of poignancy that you sense as an erotic tenderness of the heart that fills your *inner body* space.

> *Fluid flow appears when you repose in stillness long enough to give your body the time and the presence needed to engage its unfolding process.*

At first, it may feel as though this sensuous flow of *Eros* appears in particular areas in your inner body, and then it may stream to other areas. Or, you may sense a general ocean-like erotic feeling in your whole inner-body field. *Fluid consciousness* reveals how *Eros* suffuses and unites all aspects of the body that intercommunicate and convey *a felt sense* of ease, safety, trust, unity, health, and wholeness.

The mind will feel firmly settled inside the body that is united with the sensuous field that is pulsing in your *inner body space*. Your previous self-sense, which was hard-focused and concentrated, now feels expanded, buoyant, open, relaxed, spontaneous, and free-floating. As you *sensually* abide here, allow the unfolding of your fluid consciousness while the tender *Mother Love* brings your whole body to wholeness.

If the sensuous fluid flow completes itself, you may *realize* a vast expansion of your consciousness that opens into a sense of a free-fall in which your three centers of thinking, feeling, and will separate and fly apart, which feels chaotic and disorienting. See if you can relax any need to control this process due to the fear of loss. Let it deepen, if you can, and repose in *presence* without recoil so your consciousness can expand to a vast, global *Radiant Presence*.

INNER-BODY BRIGHT

In this *Radiance,* your inner body awareness expands beyond the ego's gravitational pull, and your consciousness becomes free, spacious, thin, subtle, and luminous. The tempo of your inner breathing becomes so slow that it may seem that at times there is no breath. Meanwhile, your inner body expands into a vast radiance. The mind will slow, and you realize the *Self*, which replaces the ego's sense of a separate self or 'me.' Instead, your awareness is a global field of radiance that breathes much slower, lighter, softer, quieter, and subtler, and the movements are more micro-nuanced, refined, and delicate as compared to the qualities of the fluid body breathing, which continues imperceptibly in the background. Your vast radiant breath feels like the pure awareness of the *Self*, with little or no sense of a 'me.'

Your fluid body expands and becomes a vast space that is filled with light.

After you have spent some time basking in this subtle, sensuous, micro-nuance of liquid light, which is your vastly expanded inner body, your consciousness may become more expansive and take on an empty quality. Here, in the emptiness, your perception may invert: instead of you seeing the *radiant presence*, the *loving presence* is beholding you, and you feel *loved* unconditionally, as you are. Your luminous body can be sensually characterized as the *radiant presence of love*.

You feel loved, just as you are.

DYNAMIC STILLNESS

Eventually, after a daily practice of contacting the fluid and luminous aspects of your body, your consciousness expands beyond the horizon of your known. Suddenly, your consciousness disappears into the beyond, past the known, and there is only black stillness that pervades infinite space. Meanwhile, your awareness may concentrate inwardly, become dense, which creates an inner body pressure that may feel uncomfortable. If you can bear it, your separate sense of "I" eventually disappears into a point and implodes within, which suffuses your inner body with an infinite blackness that is absolutely still.

There may be repeated cycles of this inner body implosion of black stillness into your inner body space. Each time your vast luminous body disappears and the black stillness appears, the *Self*, or pure awareness, recedes, sinks, and disappears into blackness, which becomes ever-deepening stillness, as the silent pull of Dynamic Stillness. It can feel like the awareness of the *Radiant Self* has distilled itself to a small point that finally implodes, gives out, extinguishes, and gives way. Self-consciousness disappears into an infinite velvety blackness that is awareness itself. At infinite inner stillness, all self-referencing, the sense of the *Self*, and the subtle inner breaths cease, and you become one with Absolute unmanifest Pure Consciousness.

Sometimes you return to self-consciousness from Dynamic Stillness as though you popped out of black silence like a cork that was underwater and bobbed to the surface, and you feel refreshed and whole. Other times a truth, an insight or a message from the depths will come back with you. Often there is no recollection, no memory, no sense of time, nor a sense of self at all. Even amid this *Cloud of Unknowing*, or *Divine Ignorance*, you are certain that you touched the *Mystery*. Eventually, integration occurs, and not only can you remain present in infinite stillness, your consciousness becomes an infinite *presence of stillness*.

PURE BREATH OF LOVE IS PARADOXICAL CONSCIOUSNESS

As the process deepens, infinite blackness intensifies and becomes radiant blackness, until the stillness builds in strength and becomes a powerful density. The density creates an inner body pressure that paradoxically expands your consciousness; while and at the same time, distills consciousness, which spills over the edge 'beyond infinity.' Meanwhile, the inner body pressure of the density implodes infinite consciousness inside your body, and the bottom drops out through the pelvis. You sense the *inner body* pressure of density suffuses all your cells with a liquid, blazing, lava-like quality that feels like the *Tender Mother Love* that creates all that is. If you are not accustomed to the discomfort from the inner pressure that arises from this degree of deep embodiment, it may alarm your ego, and it will want to take over control by recoiling awareness from the entire process. Ego will use all of its *Core Wound* strategies of recoil, along with practitioner recoils, ego control, diminishment, dissociation into stillness as by-pass, or, it will shut down your consciousness.[34]

If you can remain present amid the discomfort, you sense a deeply incarnating super substance that is a mysterious mix of all enfoldments and qualities of consciousness that you have previously realized, which is now combined-as-one and sealed inside infinite Dynamic Stillness.

Beyond infinity, it is as though all manifest qualities of consciousness *and* the unmanifest absolute combine and implode inside you as Dynamic Stillness. You realize that the infinitesimal point of stillness inside your cells, and the boundless outer edge of infinity, are the same place as aspects of your paradoxical consciousness.

You realize that your cumulative cellular consciousness and the *wisdom of the whole* are not separate, they are one. Paradoxical also means you can distinguish between the formless and the formed even though they are not separate. Also, you can discern that you are a limited me, *and* boundless absolute *presence of stillness*, which are seamlessly united with love that creates all that is.

You realize that beyond stillness is an ocean of love that expresses all manifest creation, and your body is the portal.

The above is a brief characterization of a meditative inner body journey of *ascent* and *descent*. *Ascent* expands your awareness beyond the control of the nervous system and egoic self-centeredness, while you realize that each element *earth, water, air, fire,* and *ether* emanate specific tonal qualities of consciousness that unite awareness with the infinite primordial *Self* of pure consciousness. Subsequently, *descent* begins as an *implosion* of consciousness of all elements that combine-as-one into the inner body infinity of Dynamic Stillness. Inside the seal of Dynamic Stillness, the body unites with love while suffusing every cell infinitesimally.

Every element of consciousness within each cell emits a unique set of luminous colors, and each color has a different frequency of vibratory tone, a luminosity, and a geometric shape which all together is a single whole.

The main point of a stillness meditative practice is the *sensing* awareness of the *Self*, in which presence is gradually stabilized and made whole in the body amid the darkness of the *Absolute Mother - The Great Black Mother*. You realize this awareness while sensing the inner body expressions of consciousness within the elements that your *sensing presence* attends to. You sense the body's unfolding *as* consciousness united with love, while you enjoy a lessening of the sense of a separate self of the ego.

You realize a gradual increase of ways that *body-as-consciousness* sensuously unfolds to its source as un-manifest stillness expressing the love that creates all that is.

I mentioned some of the spiritual traditions that consider the heart's self-existing radiance *as* a body. The Sufi's call it the *Most Sacred Body* and the *Supra Celestial Body*. It is *Rainbow Body* in Tibetan Buddhism, and *Diamond Body* or *Immortal Body* in

Taoism. Christians call it the *Resurrection Body, Glorified Body, Radiant Gloriosa, Holy Breath of Sophia,* and *Criatura.*

It is crucial that you cultivate a daily practice of *Pratyahara,* as an inward orientation of awareness while *attending to, being with,* and *sensing* the intensification of consciousness that begins as enlivening at conception to an endless journey of evolution wherein every cell awakens *as* an eternal unfolding of love.

Now we can refine our daily *Stillness Practice.*

5

REFINING YOUR DAILY STILLNESS PRACTICE

The inner reflects the outer and the outer reflects the inner.
As above, it is below.[35]

How thoroughly you navigate your inner territory determines the quality of your relationship to yourself, to others, and the world. A regular daily *Stillness Practice* strengthens your will that empowers your *presence*, which loosens the grip ego has over your attention. It is the power of your *presence* that frees you from the habitual, historical, cultural, and ancestral patterns, which create the unconscious automatic psychological complexes that become personality traits that create separation.

Your *presence* of will strengthens by a regular, daily practice of reposing inside your body space with open and free awareness. When your body's innate wisdom awakens, you spontaneously respond to life in a harmony with your *Tao*. You can then cultivate authentic responses to life that originate from your body's silent language without words that well from the depths of your embodied presence. Your bodily responses arise naturally from the spectral range of the totality of who you are, which include your hidden gifts and powers yet to be discovered until after you face your shadow.

FROM YOUR SHADOW TO YOUR PERSONAL GIFT TO YOUR TRANSPERSONAL POWER

Richard Rudd says that when your shadow is transmuted by *presence*, it alchemically returns each shadow to its original gift. Then, as you deepen your *Stillness Practice*, your unique gifts to the world transubstantiate into the transpersonal powers that the spiritual traditions call the *siddhis*.[36]

You then appreciate a spectral existence, and you express your authentic nature that includes the so-called unbearable aspects of your vast brilliant radiance, and your dreaded deep dark shadows. Once your presence of will is strong, by engaging a regular daily inner practice, you cease being moved by the ego's strategies of recoil from love to avoid the uncomfortable past, and the unbearable future. Strategies of recoil are what creates the shadow in the first place. Therefore, it is an impossible prospect for the ego to transcend the ego's control over your awareness; it is only by a strength of will that your *presence* can face and integrate your shadow. When your awareness is free, you can easily be with and express your spectral nature. When your actions spring from the wisdom of the body, it is for your good, for the good of others, and for the good of the whole. Essentially, your will yields and unites with Divine Feminine Will.

Learning to inwardly repose and sense your inner body qualities is the holy ground that unites your wisdom of the body with Divine Feminine Will. Your body then exudes an inherent wisdom that awakens you to the universal wisdom of the *Tao*.

Again, the foundational practice that connects you to the wisdom of your body is to inhabit your inner body space, and to sense with presence the tonal qualities in your inner body atmosphere, and repose here, while you let everything be *as it is*.

> *Your inner body qualities become an objective guidance in life, your GPS.*

At the core of your embodiment practice, is a trust in the inherent wisdom of your body, and a confidence that your body is connected to the natural order of the *Tao*. You can enhance your inner body wisdom and live by its guidance, when you daily receive and soak up the *presence of stillness* that dwells inside your body. This practice slows the tempo of your consciousness, so you can sense the subtle nuanced micro-qualities that pulse inside you as the inner breaths.

BODY, BREATH, TEMPO, AND THE ELEMENTS EXPRESS YOUR CONSCIOUSNESS

The body is not limited to the skin; it is an unfinished open-ended mystery made of pure consciousness and love, which is prior to the narcissistic self-serving consciousness of the ego (me). If, daily, you inwardly repose inside your body space and absorb stillness, then pure consciousness will utterly suffuse your body, psyche, and spirit. If you are fully open to let stillness suffuse your cells, they will emanate a super radiance that integrates all levels of consciousness in you that becomes love.

Differentiating which level of consciousness is predominant in you depends on the quality of the felt element, the vastness of the space of stillness that your perception has expanded into, the timing or tempo of the inner breathing of your consciousness, and the level of inclusiveness that you have self-realized.

Stillness Practices reveal five major enfoldments of consciousness, and as mentioned above, each expresses a particular space and depth of stillness in which wells an inner breath with a tempo that exudes an elemental consciousness. Your bodily experience of stillness, breath, tempo, and the elements as consciousness depends on which element is in the forefront - earth, water, air, fire, ether, or a combination of all elements. Each element expresses specific qualities of consciousness that breathe in your inner body space. The elements can also combine as one to become one quintessential element of consciousness that expresses multiple rhythms inside your body.

Below I paraphrase a beautiful translation of the Aramaic Bible.[37]

EH - FLESH - EARTH - CONSCIOUSNESS TRAPPED INSIDE THE SKIN

Eh - is a subtle Breath that is trapped in the body, self-identified, and unconnected to the slower, deeper, and vaster subtle breaths within the body.

Eh corresponds to the nervous system motion of body consciousness called the cranial wave, and its predominant element is *earth*. Earth contains the past as a holographic record of your biography that is held in the body's tissues. This breath, *Eh,* holds what is 'beneath the earth,' which is your past, your history. *Eh* represents the disposition of a life lived exclusively as a self-referencing ego that habitually lives in the past or future, and recoils consciousness from love.

Eh implies that you are in contact with, orient to, and perceive from the parts. Parts emanate the separating chaotic rhythms of the given of your body's tissues, skin, muscles, fascia, blood vessels, lymph vessels, dura, nervous system, bones, organs, anatomy, etc. In tissue consciousness, your body and awareness are under nervous system control and directed by the ego by which you feel the body as a series of separate chaotic parts that are at war. When the nervous system is in charge of your awareness, you sense a quality of dread and anxiety, which pervades because you feel separate from life. The quality inside your tissues includes unease, static, and an inner buzz.

Each inertial motion pattern in your body represents a point of dissonance between ego's narcissistic need for life to go 'my way' and the natural flow of life, the *Tao*, that is expressing life as it is.

From the Buddhist perspective, tissue consciousness expresses narcissism, which is the source of *samsara* or 'life as suffering.' Suffering expresses in the body as armor that is laid down at each point of dissonance where the ego argues with the flow of life, the *Tao*, and the ego loses the argument. Why? Because if life does not go 'my way' - the narcissistic way that ego thinks it 'should' - it triggers recoil from love as an array of self-deprecating thoughts, feelings, and emotions. You suffer from the indignities of the inner critic, and the emotions of doubt, fear, hatred, anger, shame, guilt, dread, etc. When these reactions become a habit, they form psychological complexes that trigger unsavory aspects of your personality, which create behavioral and bodily patterns that recoil you from love as a lifestyle.

Each narcissistic, self-serving emotional reaction initiates a corollary neurological stress response in the tissues that contract the ground substance, which is the liquid crystal medium for intercommunication between all the cells. Normally, the ground substance is liquid but when it contracts and turns to a gel, it blocks the fractal information that conveys wholeness to your cells that emanate from the *Tao*. The gel turns fractals into digital patterns that block the information from the blueprint of wholeness that has the vital instructions to the cells. The significant decrease in the quality of information that enters and exits the cell leads to bodily armor, behavioral patterns, symptoms, and disease that compound our suffering and brings us closer to death.

I hope it is evident that the nervous system is fundamentally reactive and is incapable of harmonizing our consciousness with the body's natural laws. Your body possesses an inherent wisdom that is far more intelligent than the nervous system that naturally synchronizes you with life and can evolve your consciousness. Fluid consciousness is the door to access your body's wisdom.

KAPH - FLUID - WATER: CONSCIOUSNESS EXPANDS TO THE SUBTLE BODY

Kaph - is a Breath of embodied *presence* that expands into and is connected to nature.

Kaph is fluid body consciousness predominated by the element of water that reveals to you *what is in the now*. Your natural state is not referenced to the past or future.

Contact with your subtle fluid body occurs when your consciousness expands beyond egoic narcissism and is freed from the nervous system's control of the body. The fluid body reveals the wisdom of the body as a uniting principle that interconnects the body with the mind. The bodymind directly accesses the wisdom of nature, the *Sophia*, or Soul. Your expanded consciousness realizes the fluidic expressions of life; it is no longer under the control of the nervous system or the ego, which dissolves the narcissistic restrictions placed upon the boundless expressive flow of the *Tao*.

Therefore, we realize that the wisdom of the body is inherent to fluid consciousness. Contractions in the body self-resolve whenever we attend to them with presence. Your felt-sense in the fluid consciousness is of an elegant, soothing, sensuous, even erotic, fluid flow as a rhythm that joyously returns gelled, contracted ground substance into a fluid again. Thus, the wounds of suffering from the past that are stored as armor in the body, are synchronized with the *presence of stillness* and the body begins its journey to become whole. When the practice of fluid consciousness bears fruit and integrates, your consciousness expands to a vast Radiant Presence that is the template of wholeness.

HETH - VAST LUMINOUS VAPOR - AIR AND FIRE: GLOBAL CONSCIOUSNESS

Heth - is a subtle Breath that is non-personal, a luminous body-as-consciousness.

Heth is a mix of elements *air and fire*, expressed as vast luminescence. *Radiant Presence* is your *Self*, a unified consciousness that evolves you toward your destiny, and expresses your essence.

You enjoy body-felt contact with your archetypal *Self* after the fluid body has self-resolved a sufficient number of points of contractions in the body, which opens your core midline. When your midline or central channel opens, stillness fills your body, the room, and the biosphere, and you receive a global suffusion of a vast Radiant Presence that co-breathes in you as the Unified Consciousness of the *Self*. This is a transpersonal realization that leads to becoming whole. In essence, you realize the Archetypal *Self* that comes from the future to meet with your 'given' of the past, and the present that is now. The *Self*, on a deeper level, is one with Source. Jung calls this realization the *Purusha*, a vedic term that translates to 'Godman.'[38] You enjoy global unified consciousness by which you realize your life's destiny; the 'why' you came to earth becomes so obvious that you can now fully live your life while you are being lived by the Divine Will.

After you bodily acclimate to this unified consciousness that expresses as your vast luminous *Self*, there comes the point at which the ego surrenders its need to control life, which will also free your body from nervous system control by which your suffering will end. This is when you realize a body-felt contact with infinite stillness that is pure consciousness, or Dynamic Stillness.

HEY - DYNAMIC STILLNESS - QUINTESSENTIAL ETHER: INFINITE CONSCIOUSNESS

Hey - is a highly refined Breath unencumbered and free from the notion of a limited physical body.

Hey is Dynamic Stillness, the quintessential substance of *ether*. A timeless, infinitely spacious domain that is prior-to a consciousness that is oriented to a self or *Self*.

This is a realization of a timeless, self-identity-less, boundless, and position-less domain. You know your consciousness is an expression of the Consciousness of the Whole without knowing how you know. Some non-dual traditions consider this realization to be the end-all and be all on the path of self-realization. Yet, if you choose to continue your journey to evolve consciousness, this stage becomes a portal that leads to freedom. Beyond Stillness, all prior levels of consciousness that you have realized unite inside you and become the *Pure Breath of Love*.

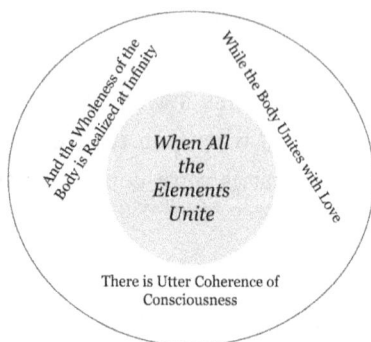

When All
the
Elements
Unite

And the Wholeness of the Body is Realized at Infinity

While the Body Unites with Love

There is Utter Coherence of
Consciousness

Figure 4. When All the Elements Unite

After Dynamic Stillness becomes your perception, your infinite consciousness gradually 'lands' inside every cell in your body. This is an utter embodiment of infinite stillness that is accompanied by an unimpeded suffusion of *Pure Breath of Love* in all your cells. Each cell Radiantly Awakens with a consciousness that emanates to infinity and back to the body. You can no longer discern or sense separation anywhere. This depth of utter, embodied realization of the cells is known as enfleshment.

It is important to distinguish between enfleshment and an encounter with the empty void that terrifies the ego. Because the ego is a self-reflective consciousness, when it dissolves it becomes filled with dread, wondering where 'I' went, and what is going to happen now that the narcissistic self-serving 'me' is gone. Even a brief contact with this terror, due to an egoic mis-identification with the empty void, prevents many people from crossing over to freedom.[39]

In a disembodied non-duality, the ego 'thinks' emptiness is reality, so it separates itself from the body saying "I am not my body." However, the opposite realization occurs when every

84

cell awakens in an utter union with the love that creates all that is.

Body is the love that creates all that is.

Engaging our *Stillness Practice* is challenging because ego intensely avoids self-development. Also, we have a major threshold to cross. Namely, ego's greatest terror, which is to bear the unbearable pain of the *Core Erotic Wound*, or *Grail Wound*, and to navigate all the hidden physical and psychological complexes that unconsciously recoil our awareness from love. Recall that the *Core Erotic Wound* is an event in our life that is so traumatic it separates us from a body-felt connection with *Eros*, the life force that powers our will. This leads us to explore practices to balance the feminine and masculine dynamics.

The rest of this chapter was created by students during a Muir Beach, CA *Mentor Course* in 2008.

HOW FEMININE AND MASCULINE PRINCIPLES OPERATE IN HARMONY

NOTE: The feminine and the masculine principles are polar forces that exist in the bodies of both genders in varying degrees. When you do not project your desire onto an object to fulfill your ego's needs, and instead you hold desire inside, then the Feminine Wisdom guides you. Furthermore, when desire is held in unconditional regard, that is the Positive Masculine, which when harmonized with feminine desire ignites the inner marriage. Here are some of the manifestations of the marriage.

The positive feminine meets all negative aspects, both the masculine and feminine, relationally with tenderness, caring, and love. She is matter, the body, sensuality, feelings, sexuality, intensity, darkness, mother earth, and love expressed.

The positive masculine is conscious space, head centered and filled with the light of presence with an ability to be unflinchingly present, conscious, and non-conditional. He is unwaveringly *present* to the negative masculine *and* to the negative feminine.

In a nutshell:

- Wholeness is the ability to be consciously aware (positive masculine) and in relationship (positive feminine) with *anything* that happens.
- Sutherland's version of wholeness: to be in synchronicity with all fulcrums.

REWIRING

Developing an unconditional presence to *be-with* is an ability to tolerate relationships from the disposition of *"don't know" "don't understand,"* amid a *trust in the process* as it unfolds moment by moment. Innocence and trust cleanse the limbic system and rewires the nervous system. In the *presence of stillness*, there is more space while time slows; therefore, it is easier to be *present* due to levity. The more gravity, the more rapid the tempo, and the more difficult it is to be present due to the increased speed that produces greater intensity. Levity is realized by dropping into the inner body space that has a slower tempo than the mind, as a positive masculine act of consciousness.

The slowing down of presence allows a savoring of the nuances that arise as inner body qualities: this is intimacy with self, which allows us to remain in an unflinching *presence of stillness*. This practice unites the positive masculine and feminine that becomes a path to the inner marriage of body-as-consciousness that expresses love. However, the patriarchal disposition impedes the sacred inner marriage.

THE PATRIARCHAL HATRED AND TERROR OF THE FEMININE PRINCIPLE

The major impediment to an inner marriage between the feminine and masculine forces within us is a patriarchal disposition, which is filled with hatred and terror of feminine power, and this infects the bodies of men and women. The brain-driven hypermasculine disposition has controlled *Eros*, the *Shakti*, in women's bodies for many generations.

One result is that the feminine suffers the *wound of silence:*

> *An inability to speak up and ask for your heart's longing and your body's desire.* To reverse this ancient wound inflicted on the feminine by the dominating hypermasculine patriarchy, practice expressing your *wisdom voice.*

PRACTICES TO ENHANCE THE FEMININE PRINCIPLE: ACTIVATE YOUR WISDOM VOICE AND ASK FOR WHAT YOU WANT

To reconnect with your *wisdom voice,* attune *inside* your lower pelvis, and *sense* the waves of *Eros* that pulse as fractal expressions of *Shakti* inside your flesh. Allow the tonal quality of these sensuous pulses to guide you in your choices, your words, your body's movements and actions without letting the ego edit or interfere with *Shakti's* subtle guidance. Let love, or *Shakti* move your body as a sacred tenderness of Divine Feminine Will.

The quiet tenderness of Mother Love replaces the harsh, fear-based negative masculine guidance that can become cruel bodily treatment and deprivation due to a sense of un-deservability, which can also drive your choices, actions, and movements. All this is derived from patriarchal energies that are trapped in the flesh. Signs of the hypermasculine include bodily armor, intense emotions, rapidly changing moods, weakened will, low vital energy, repeated illnesses that deplete the immune system, an inability to confront conflict or intensity, difficulty with commitment or follow through, fear to ask for what your heart desires, and an inability to realize and manifest your life purpose. When hypermasculine control of the body exhausts the will, it can lead to a collapse into the hyperfeminine disposition. Hyperfeminine tendencies manifest as cruel mistreatment of the body, extreme diets, fasting, and enemas, that can become eating disorders, deprivation, or over exercise, etc. The power of your *Eros*, your will, as the bodily expression of love, can become so depleted that it is uncomfortable to be in the body, so dissociation is common. When the free-flow of *Shakti* is blocked in the body, it diminishes your body's sublime expressions of the Tender Mother Love.

To transmute the ancient patriarchal *wound of silence,* spend time daily sitting in stillness inside your womb space, while you practice *Pratyahara:* attend *inside* the space of your womb and contact the sensuous waves of your heart's longing, and let your *inner* desire lead your body. This is the opposite of the snake, which is guided by the projected desires of ego to get from others for selfish gain. Instead, inner desire evolves consciousness to wholeness.[40]

Let your body move and be guided by your heart's inner longing while your body's desire wells as the *Shakti,* the *Eros* from your womb, which is the source of your *wisdom voice.*

Shakti is *Kundalini,* the Sacred Force of Love, so do not second guess, override, or edit your heart's longing for a bodily union with love. *Shakti* softly leads you to a deep bodily intimacy as you let your inner, still, quiet, delicate inner longing speak up, by *asking* for what *body* desires. *Ask* bodily with your body's subtle gestures that express *Shakti,* as she guides you deeper into intimacy as a bodily union with love.

Ask for what you want as it wells in subtle quiet waves of *inner* desire that softly pulse in your womb. Again, this aspect of bodily desire evolves consciousness as a subtle pulse from *within* your womb's flesh. Let its subtle longing for bodily union with love be in charge of what you ask for, your body's motions, your choice of a partner, and your actions in life. The Tender Love of the Divine Feminine Will suffuses your cells and your body becomes Love.

Again, your subtle heart's longing, as inner bodily desire, arises as sensuous pulsing waves *inside* your womb. Remain attuned to *Eros* and stay with your arousal, which expresses the quiet longing of your wombs' *inner desire for union.* Let *Shakti* guide you - as you hold the desires of your body *inside*, letting them implode as the tenderest inner-body expressions of love that move your body.

One aspect of a practice that strengthens the feminine principle is to maintain a constant *inner* contact with arousal that wells as an inner longing that pulses as subtle bodily desire for union with the tenderest bodily expressions of love.

Orient to the desire *inside you,* and do not project it out; this practice builds the potency of *innate bliss.* Then *innate bliss* guides you bodily to ask for what you long for, as it arises as *waves of desire from within. Shakti* will guide your body's motions, instead of being driven by the ego and the snake that is based on history, shadow, and the over-exuberant animal impulse from the nervous system to get from an object for selfish gain. Engaging this practice cultivates discernment between what arises from the nervous system-driven ego that is oriented to personal gratification, and the soft, quiet inner longing of the heart that is bodily desire that is one with the Tender Mother Love, the greatest healing force on earth. *Prajnaparamita* is for the good of the whole.

This sacred feminine practice builds confidence, wisdom, and strength of will in a *Shakti* empowered female. *Inwardly* sense the subtle pulsing waves of desire in your womb space and *Shakti* will guide your body.

You do not secretly expect an outcome, dare to ask.

Once you bodily soften, open, and can abide in a deep repose with the *Shakti*, which is already one with love, you can trust her soft, quiet, inner guidance. She'll take care of boundaries, safety, and containment while the Tender Mother Love provides the embodied ground that cultivates Love's full blossoming *in your every cell* until your body is love. Love in freedom means "not my will, but it is the tender Divine Feminine Love that guides my body and my psyche."

MAN AND WOMAN MUTUALLY BREAK THE OLD PATTERNS TOGETHER

It may be challenging to take responsibility as a *Shakti* empowered being by asking for what you want, because the hypermasculine patriarchy has dominated female and male bodies for many generations.

POTENT PRACTICE FOR THE FEMININE

Again, if you desire to directly express your *Shakti* empowerment, bodily ask for what *the feminine* desires. Then your body's motions will express *her* heart's longing even <u>while *she*</u> experiences shadow, fear, mistrust, or ego-driven strategies that control intimacy, and amid intense arousal. This *practice of presence* amid intensity, intimacy, or paradox opens the body into the utter depths of love. Your open-hearted bodily repose, while in a *felt-contact* with your heart's longing as guided by the pelvic pulse, is a path for bodily expressing *Shakti*'s desire. Practice this *while* you feel the shadows of fear, doubt, hatred, lack of trust, holding back, guilt, shame, suspicion, control, recoil, armor, recoil, arousal, orgasm, love, ... see if you can include everything.

PRACTICE FOR THE MASCULINE

A masculine can support a feminine practice by learning to wait until *she* asks. The masculine utilizes *Pratyahara* by orienting inwardly into stillness as pure consciousness (*Shiva*) while reposing inside in an unwavering presence to wait ... until asked by the *Shakti* to serve her as she is moved by her pelvic wisdom. This rebalances the relationship between *Shakti* and *Shiva*. Again, the masculine does not initiate, but waits until asked bodily by the feminine. When she asks bodily for what she desires from the heart, as it arises from the longing within her sacred pulse, he serves her if he is able. *Inner desire* is expressed bodily as the soft pulsing waves of *Eros within the body*. The masculine does not push or guide the intimacy process, he responds to the wisdom of a woman's bodily guidance that wells from within as the *Shakti*.

BODY AS SOUL

When free, desire in a woman pulses as erotic waves from within her womb as her inner heart's desire *in her body*. This guides the movements of her body even amid a daunting shadow, intensity, emotions, memories, fear, holding back, bodily recoil, armor, and any degree of intimacy or paradox that she encounters. All this energy - the most dreaded horror of the shadow and the unbearable Radiance of Love - dissolves into the *presence of stillness* as pure consciousness. When stillness deeply incarnates into the flesh, the body pulses as tender soft *Eros* that wells from within the womb and moves the body as sensuous waves of Love throughout all cells: this is the *body-felt* sensation when the presence of the *Shakti* is united with the cells in a woman's body. *Shakti* as Soul transmutes the body into *Criatura,* the sacred being of love endowed with a cat-like sensuous freedom as her body's expression.

> *Criatura* is born when the *Sacred Pulse of Love* awakens in the *womb-heart.*

When a woman can feel the sensuous waves pulsing inside the flesh of her womb, the *Shakti* is present and she can trust that the wisdom of the *Spanda* guides her desire and the motions of her body because it comes from love. She navigates deeper into intimacy regardless of shadow, fear, lack of trust, armor, bodily holding back, lack of vitality, recoil, control strategies, snake's antics, etc., because she lets *Spanda* guide her body's tender expressions.

> *Shakti* is in charge and guides, while *Shiva* serves.

Recall that *Stillness Touch* is rooted in the ancient tantric spiritual practice of Kashmir Shaivism. One aspect of this practice is to be aware that any touch you offer is without a subject or an object. There is no agenda, goal, or a need for any outcome: it is a free-will offering. All there is to 'do' is orient inside and sense the *Sacred Pulse of the Spanda* and let it guide your body while love moves your flesh.

Stillness Touch is a potent path for embodying love that can return your body to its original state as a Sacred Vessel of Love, the *Criatura.* When you are in contact with *inner desire* connected to wisdom it cultivates a continuity of consciousness that frees attention, which naturally leads you deeper into intimacy - all based on your *felt-sense* of the inner pulsing waves that well from your womb's flesh as they arise from *Shakti*.

Another helpful practice is to bodily soften and repose inwardly in contact with love, instead of being controlled by nervous system ego-driven karma, history, thoughts, ideas, lack of energy, not feeling like it, excuses, and the worn out fears derived from shadow, or due to the patriarchal control strategies that drive the snake's antics, which confess a misuse of the *Kundalini*, the Sacred Force of Love. The snake uses the nervous system and our history to drive the body, which creates armor that recoils awareness away from a bodily union with love. Instead, repose *inside* the sacred space of your womb, and let your heart's pulse open a gateway to erotic stillness in freedom as guided by the Tender Mother Love. The following traits were crafted by students in a 2007 Muir Beach, CA Mentor Course.

POSITIVE FEMININE TRAITS (APPLIES TO BOTH SEXES)

The positive feminine knows that her body is *Criatura*, the quintessential expression of love, and she is in continuous contact with her wisdom voice.

- A positive feminine trait is to feel love for the individual, the parts, and the whole all at once.
- She emanates love for all that is in an inclusive way: love of the one and the many.
- She desires connection, relatedness, union, and wholeness.
- She strives for harmony, health, and evolution.
- She can relate deeply to the body, the sensual and erotic, and she is not afraid to express them.
- She accepts the movement of her will as the flow of desire that is guided by the wisdom of the body.

- She is empathetic and feels the other and compassionately accepts who they are unconditionally.
- Before taking action, she takes into account the good of the whole.

NEGATIVE FEMININE TRAITS (APPLIES TO BOTH SEXES)

When we shut down desire or project it out onto objects, this hinders authentic physical feelings, which represses *Eros*, which will then turn into mysterious illnesses of all sorts. Physical, mental, psychological, and spiritual symptoms express as various forms of bodily self-harm, distorted body self-image, self-hatred, self-violent communications of the inner critic, dissociation, confusion, disdain toward ever-changing chaotic moods, inner instability, restlessness, lack of ground, irritability, incapacity to be with intensity because it erodes the sense of ground or center.

A woman's flesh is absorptive, so she not only has typical negative feminine traits, she can also become infected by aspects of the negative hypermasculine. This imbalance harms sexuality and creates misperceptions such as, 'sex is evil' or we become a prude, a manipulative teaser, a sexual predator, a corporate hard-ass, or can act out hatred for the masculine by displaying more negative masculine! One student confessed that in her youth she would dress up as a man and go to bars to pick fights with men. This manifests the cheapest part of the negative masculine that can be expressed in a woman's body and psyche.

- A classic negative feminine shadow is called the *fiendess*, who displays fits of uncontrolled emotionality that threaten the masculine in ways that ignite castration terror. Instead of taking care of his own needs, he becomes her slave. A typical response toward the fiendess is, "Yes dear" because the fiendess is, "She who must be obeyed."

- A woman stuck in the negative feminine can be engulfing, devouring, insatiable, and unable to discern appropriate boundaries.
- She can fall too deeply into the manifest without remaining in connection to her inner-body guidance. For example, she is unable to see ahead and take into account the impact her actions may have on others.
- She is over-involved in others' business, and in God's business.
- She wants you to be the way she wants you to be, yet is unable to tell you what it is she wants, and if you don't give it to her, she withdraws, withholds relatedness, or cuts off sexual connection in its varied forms and hurts you emotionally, physically, or spiritually to punish you.
- She can be over emotional, explosive, mocking, cutting, and hateful.
- Unable to keep agreements, and is unreliable.
- Teases, mis-uses her 'cunt power' to get what she wants: a job, social status, husband, the various perks of life, etc.
- Mocks, fears, or demonizes the masculine animal drive for procreation, yet wants and needs him anyway, and then she is angry at herself for collapsing to be used by him, which is projected as hatred onto the man.
- Unable to trust a man, or *herself*, because she is afraid of her own inner power and does not trust it.
- Stirs up rumors and falsehoods, bad mouths others, and enacts self-victimhood.

POSITIVE MASCULINE TRAITS (APPLIES TO BOTH SEXES)

- Boundaries, the ability to say no in order to say yes, are important.
- With boundaries, we can discern when to say, "slow down" or "stop."
- On the other side, when the feminine sets a boundary the positive masculine is fierce about not pushing the edges that violate the safety envelope that she set.
- Positive masculine says to the feminine: "There is room for you to be exactly who you are, and I will be present to your process."
- Action takes everything into account for the good of the whole, is a fierce *guardian for the other and the whole.*
- Is willing to *consciously* sacrifice some of himself for the person who has shown him their un-tarnished gold. In a *Stillness Touch* session this manifests as a willingness to co-resonate with the recipient; to 'suffer with' an open heart helps the recipient metabolize intensity, intimacy, and paradox that vibrates through their and our inner body space.
- Positive masculine does not need to talk, yet there is a commitment to be the guardian of the Gold by offering an unconditional space for any and all manifestations. This creates the free space for the feminine to express.
- Discernment: remain mindful of being inside stillness to 'down-tempo' awareness to discern 'yes' or 'no' in each moment.
- The call to consciousness is to be aware of automaticity as a re-enactment of the past, amid too-much comfort, and to not be detoured by intensity, exuberance, or the inflation of enthusiasm that pushes us to rush to the future: these are indications of 'slow down' or 'no.'

- A healthy ability to say this is fake.
- To be present in an appropriate way to the negative masculine and can guard against the inner critic taking control, by virtue of the wisdom of discernment – ability to be humorous, and without charge to recognize when the inner critic is present: 'there you go again'. This disposition of unconditional regard applies to all our so-called negative traits, feminine or masculine.

NEGATIVE MASCULINE TRAITS (APPLIES TO BOTH SEXES)

A man possessed by excessive negative female traits is the classic new age man:

emasculated, castrated, overly soft, sweet, and inappropriately surrenders himself to serve the woman as self-betrayal: 'whatever you want, dear.' He does not have the strength to be present to a woman when she is displeased, moody, or emotional. He `can be seen on the dance floor dancing like a woman. He is winey, a victim, unable to take a stand, wavers, unable to make decisions or to commit, unable to speak up, unable to discern: 'It's all good.' He is incapable of fierceness even when it is appropriate.

- Lack of presence.
- Withdrawing, dismissive, looks down upon, irritated.
- Getting-using-manipulating-coercing, dominating, controlling.
- Measuring and comparing: "You'll never measure up."
- Non-relational, unless there is something for him 'to get' out of it that is of use.
- Objectifying, therefore, separating.
- Does not take everything into account, is out for

himself, protects and defends *against the other,* and *everything* is other!

- "You're bad, you're broken, you are an adversary"
- Inner critic: "You're doing it wrong. You're no good."
- Is 'me'- driven, and excessively motivated by his hypermasculine 'testosterone animal' (For example, a male deer will kill a female doe during mating season).
- The earth's resources are here to be used, exploited, etc. The USA National Park motto: 'Land of many uses.'
- Nature's forces will be outsmarted, conquered, and placed into our service; an example is the medical profession's belief in conquering disease and overcoming death.

We have mentioned many aspects of the *Grail Wound,* which we will now thoroughly explore in the next two chapters.

6

OWNING YOUR GRAIL WOUND, PART 1

Great master Sri Aurobindo, emphasized the descending current as a path for the evolution of consciousness. Descent means that we journey *inside our body* to face our shadow. Below, Sri Aurobindo sets the tone for *Owning Your Grail Wound,*

"Evolution does not move higher and higher, into an ever more heavenly heaven, but deeper and deeper. Each evolutionary cycle closes a little lower, a little nearer to the Center where the supreme High and Low, heaven and earth, will finally meet. The pioneer must therefore clear up the intermediary mental, vital, and material levels so that the two poles can actually meet. When the joining takes place, not only mentally and vitally but also materially, then the Spirit will emerge in Matter within a complete supramental being and a supramental body. The difficulties of accustoming the body to the supramental Agni may, ultimately, have a reason and a purpose.

All obstacles, whatever their nature, always ultimately prove themselves to be helpful auxiliaries of a Truth whose meaning and purpose we do not yet know. To our outer, superficial vision, the transformation seems to be exclusively a physical problem, because we always put the cart before the horse, but all difficulties are actually inner and psychological; the visible and dramatic difficulties of the body's growing accustomed to the boiling Agni may be, as we shall see, less a practical or material problem than one involving the whole terrestrial consciousness.

If a pygmy were abruptly subjected to the simple mental light of an educated man, it would probably cause in the poor fellow subterranean revolutions that would traumatize him forever and drive him insane. There is still too much jungle underneath. This present world is still full of jungles: such is the problem in a nutshell. Our mental colonization is a very thin crust over a barely dried Stone Age.

Night after night, in his sleep or with his eyes wide open, the seeker uncovers very strange worlds. One after another, he unearths all the birthplaces of human perversion, human wars, human concentration camps, where everything we live here is being prepared; he catches all the sordid forces that move the petty and cruel men.

The more Light he possesses, the more darkness he uncovers. Night after night he tracks down the surreptitious rot that undermines Life; for how can anything change as long as that gangrene is there?

Now the dark half of the truth has become illuminated. Every stumbling or error kindles a flame of pain and seems to produce a breach of light below; every weakness summons up a corresponding force, as if the energy of the fall were the very energy of the ascent; every imperfection is a step toward a greater fulfillment. There are no sins, no errors, but only countless mishaps that compel us to attend to the full extent of our kingdom and to embrace everything in order to heal and fulfill everything. Through a tiny crack in our armor, a love and compassion for the world have entered in, which none of the radiant purities can ever understand; purity is impregnable, self-contained, sealed off like a fortress; some fissure is needed for the Truth to come in!

There is a truth of Love behind evil. The nearer one draws to the infernal circles, the more one uncovers the great need in the depths of Evil and begins to understand that nothing can be healed without a corresponding intensity: a flame is kindled within, more and more powerful and warm beneath the suffocating pressure – there is just Her, nothing but Her – as if Love alone could confront the Night and persuade it of its luminous half.

As if all that Shadow had been necessary so that Love might be born. In truth, the heart of every shadow, of every evil harbors the inverse mystery. And as each of us bears or harbors a special difficulty, at once the contradiction and the sign of our destiny, it may be that, similarly, the immense "faults" of the earth – her sins and sufferings and the thousand gaping wounds of a pauper – are the very sign of her destiny, and that someday she will incarnate perfect Love and Joy because she will have suffered all and understood all.

As we progress, the superconscious line recedes upward and the subconscious line downward. Everything widens, everything is illuminated, but everything also closes in and converges around a sharp point of darkness, increasingly acute, crucial and pressing, as if we had turned for years and years – for lifetimes – around the same Problem without ever having truly touched it.

Then, suddenly, it is right there, at the bottom of the hole, wriggling beneath the Light - all the evil of the world within one point.

The time of the Secret is drawing near. For the law of descent is not a law of oppression, sin, or fall, any more than it is a law of repentance or heavenward escape, but truly a Golden Law, an unfathomable Premeditation that draws us simultaneously upward and downward into the depths of the subconscient and inconscient, to that central point, that knot of life and death, shadow and light, where the Secret awaits us. The nearer we draw to the Summit, the more we touch the Depths."[41]

Please digest descending current master Sri Aurobindo's characterization of the human condition. He points out that we each bear our special difficulty, the *Grail Wound,* that is at once the contradiction and the sign of our destiny. Also, he notes that our greatest terror is facing the nearly unbearable pain of the core evil that guards the threshold to a bodily union with love. What's more, although Sri Aurobindo did not mention it by name, what he calls the 'problem' is the ego's lifelong vow:

> "I will never again feel the pain of the core evil that was created by the *Grail Wound.*"

If we desire to *know thyself,* it means to bear owning our *Grail Wound,* which opens us to the realization of the perennial inquiry that guards the initiate threshold:

"For Whom Does the Grail Serve?"

> *The Grail is Divine Feminine Will, which is the love*
> *that creates all that is.*
> *The Grail is the inside of the inside of the universal*
> *creative force of love.*
> Eros *is your will that can choose to unite your*
> *consciousness with Divine Will.*
> *The Grail Castle is your body overflowing with* Eros
> *and united with love.*

WHAT IS THE GRAIL WOUND?

As tender innocent youths, we enjoyed an unbroken erotic bodily union with love; then an overwhelmingly painful event occurred: a parent, loved one or another delivered a wound so excruciating it severed our body-felt connection with *Eros*. In depth-psychology this event is called the *Core Erotic Wound*.

> The trauma of the *Core Erotic Wound* split us from our *Eros* and created ego, as the sense of separation from love, which marked our fall from Grace. After suffering the *Core Erotic Wound*, our will was subjugated by the ego and placed under the control of narcissistic complexes that formed our personality.

When the ego only serves itself, it is known as the snake.

> *"For whom does the Grail serve?" The snake's answer is "**me**."*

It takes profound courage of heart to face the horrifying reality that we suffer from the effects of *Core Erotic Wound*. *Eros*, our will, no longer belongs to us, and we feel disconnected from the Divine Feminine Will. Instead of love, the psychological complexes direct the ego to misuse our will to do the snake's bidding for selfish gain.

The snake is a decadent form of the *Kundalini*, the great serpent power that lies coiled in the sacrum at Chakra 2 that when free rises to the heart radiance, becomes conscious and emanates the *Sacred Force of Love* that unites all things.

> *Whenever ego misuses our Eros for selfish gain, it is the work of the snake.*

It is harrowing to admit that our parents, relatives, friends, beloveds, neighbors and even strangers inflicted upon us the

Core Erotic Wound when we were tender, innocent youths. More difficult to bear is that we, in turn, act out the snake's antics and inflict the core wound on others. The *Core Erotic Wound*, which is another name for the *Grail Wound*, was handed down along our multi-generational ancestral bloodline to our parents. Then our mother, father, siblings, relatives, caregivers and loved ones unwittingly behaved in ways that so traumatized us we lost our body-felt connection with *Eros*. By acts of omission or commission - something they said or did or did not say or do - cut off our body-felt contact with love.

> *The Grail Wound creates personality traits that we struggle with life-long. The core sense of separation from Eros marks a personal beginning of suffering, having lost our natural body-felt union with love.*

To face our *Core Erotic Wound* means that we feel the full impact it has on us; this is the first step of a slow, long, painful journey to integrate life-long dysfunctional behavior patterns that block us from freely opening our body to love. When we are free from the psychological complexes that misuse our *Eros*, then by recognition, presence, and overcoming our denial of them, love will express our creative, generative life force.

> *Eros,* when freed from narcissistic ego's control, naturally reunites with love.

DENIAL AS SELF-CONDEMNATION

If we deny that we received a *Core Erotic Wound*, or we insist that it healed, we deprive ourselves of the opportunity to build the required strength of will by feeling the excruciating impact it has on our lives and others. In denial, we face the prospect that we will suffer the *Grail Wound* and remain a prisoner to our complexes life-long.

HISTORY OF THE GRAIL WOUND

The name *Grail Wound* comes from the German myth *Parzival and the Fisher King.* This ancient Western myth depicts a king wounded in his groin, the creative, generative, vital second chakra area. Paralyzed in his will leaves the king unable to act and rule the kingdom. The *Grail Wound* also reflects the parable in the Bible that describes a man paralyzed for thirty-eight years, lying in a bed by the healing fountain in Bethesda. When Christ came upon him and asked the man if he wanted to get well, the man said that there is no one to help him go to the water. Christ told the man to 'take up your bed and walk.' And so he did. Like the paralyzed man and the wounded Fisher King, it is our task to resurrect our paralyzed will by taking up the bed of our *given,* and walk.

KNOW THYSELF, RESURRECTION, UTTER UNION OF BODY AND LOVE

Self-resurrection calls for a courageous heart of presence and the profound humility to recognize, face, feel, own, confess and integrate the unbearably painful feelings, emotions, and behavioral patterns that we suffer due to the *Grail Wound.* We also take responsibility for our selfish behaviors by facing the way we treat ourselves and others. These are the preliminary steps that lead us to the threshold that we must cross all alone. The path to utter freedom from acting out the snake, if we are sufficiently fierce-hearted and we possess the courage to *know thyself,* is to muster the alchemy of presence to *unite with our snake patterns.* This is your walk, no one can do it for you.

This radical act frees attention, and *Eros* automatically reunites with love. Again, for self-resurrection, our final task is to *unite* our presence with it all.

THE PATH OF EROS

When *Eros* becomes trapped in our flesh, it lays down patterns of body armor that exhibit emotion-laden recoiling, defensive behaviors that block *Eros,* drains our vitality, passion, and creativity, and extinguishes our longing to evolve. Uniting our presence with the *Core Erotic Wound* frees *Eros*, which reverses all these effects.

> *Eros is our will, the creative desire to fulfill our destiny in all spheres of our life.*

Eros is our authentic personal power, an aspect of the Divine Feminine power of love that makes the body, heals the body, maintains the body, and evolves our consciousness. *Eros* powers our attention so love can guide our thoughts, feelings, emotions, speech, and actions. *Eros* gives us our strength of will to surrender and unite our body with love, ... or not, depending on if our *Eros* belongs to us, or to the snake.

One simple act of will that liberates your *Eros* from ego's clutches is orient inward with free attention, repose in stillness, while you sense the qualities of the sensations within you. Now let's dive into how the snake controls our *Eros.*

OBJECTIFICATION CREATES A FALSE SENSE OF SEPARATION

In our essence, everything is united; there is no separation in reality. Objectification is the portal to the duality that creates ego's false *sense of separation* that contrives a subject *me* and an object *you*. The ego objectifies, drives our attention outward toward an object, while narcissistic thinking directs the will to *get from* you because you are an object for my use. Objects that the ego designates for our misuse can be any person (including a client), a situation, a circumstance, a psychological construct, a job position, or a thing.

When we operate from the ego's false sense of separation and its narcissism, then whatever we think, feel, say, and do becomes a strategy to *get from* people and situations. In essence, everything is here to serve us and fulfill our selfish desires.

Any act of the will that comes from the narcissistic ego creates suffering.

Objectification ends when we engage the ancient practice of *Pratyahara*, which is orienting inwardly with free attention while you sense the divinity that resides inside. Opposite to that, by objectification and orienting attention outward, you live imprisoned in the duality of a narcissistic ego's false projection of separation. To permanently reverse ego's dualistic perspective, you regularly practice orienting awareness inward, and with free attention sense the qualities therein. When innerness bears fruit, it ignites the Divine Feminine principle that automatically reunites 'subject' and 'object' - the *two become one*. Once you connect inwardly to the *presence of stillness*, your attention joins with the one substance of love, and artificial separation ends. Recall that this uniting principle in which the two become one is called *Sophia*, and the practice of orienting awareness inward is *Pratyahara*.

Everything is love, and nothing is separate from it. When the ego misperceives this reality, it fragments your consciousness.

If you remain inside and present to sense the qualities within, you automatically connect to what the Buddhists call *innate bliss*, which is the natural bliss of the wisdom of the body, or *prajna*. Christians call this inner body wisdom the *Sophia*. Reconnecting to *prajna* or *Sophia* reunites all fragmented aspects of consciousness and reconnects them to the Wisdom of the Whole, the *Prajnaparamita*.

Unfortunately, without a regular daily practice of *Pratyahara*, we prolong the suffering of the *Grail Wound* and fall under the influence of its shadow, the snake. Under the snake's influence, we feel separated from our original *Edenic State* of being in a bodily union with love. I paraphrase below a brilliant character-ization of our fall from grace that is written from a Christian perspective.

> The Wholeness of life and love spontaneously flows through us as young children; we are transparent to and connected with the Kingdom of Heaven. It is a fact; both embryology and child psychology validate this truth. It is inwardly obvious. We are all created and live inside a polarity of two opposing forces, the Perfect and the conditional. The Perfect Whole is united with Love, and the imperfect, conditional part separates from love.

> In esoteric Christian language, we live a conditional life when we live exclusively from the energies of *The Fall*. To restore our original state that existed before *The Fall*, we must reestablish our conscious relationship with the love that is whole and is prior-to our ancestral genetics. Our attention needs to be free again: to naturally freely flow to love, rather than being trapped in the conditional prison. The conditional forces are in our DNA, inside the cell nucleus we inherited from our ancestral-genetic lineage of our fathers and mothers. These forces are the effect of the fall from Divine Grace that is passed on from generation to generation.

The forces of genetics have a profound power over us as the primary control of our behavior and sensory experience.

Because parents raise children in their own image to be just like them, they transmit to children their fears, attitudes toward the feminine, body, sexuality, and their disposition toward life. Parents cannot see their children as they are and love them as such. The result of being raised in the image of our parents is we get caught-up and controlled by the flow of all their limitations from their ancestors and culture, and we have only occasional glimpses of contact with the Freedom of love.

We may be caught in the flow of the culture and are either unaware or get only occasional glimpses of The Silent Night of Heaven. Anyone who has met Christ, Mary, the Holy Spirit has the deep desire to reconnect to the perfect. But our connection with love comes and goes and feels unstable, and love often feels so far away. This illusion arises from our genetics: as our ancestral and cultural influences that are more clever than us. We actually believe that these genetic family influences are real; they are, but they are not our true birthright.

These illusory ancestral forces that we inherited from our family fix our attention so it cannot flow freely towards the Beloved, towards the ocean of our home, to love. Fixation of our attention by our familial forces inhibits in us the healthy freedom of the motion of love. When the flow of the attention is free, it naturally flows to love. Love is what keeps our senses fresh, alive, vital, and leads to wholeness.

This is love in freedom.

If your blood did not flow easily, you would become ill. The free-flow of your attention is also vital to your health. When attention flows as it was intended toward love, we feel life as an ever-changing river filled with Grace. This is normal! But when we are constricted and fixed, we are asleep to the flow of love, and we are full of fears and personal beliefs, so we are weary and can find no rest. The flow of our attention determines what our senses perceive; we manipulate our attention so much that we end up tired and weary. When our attention is left alone - free - it automatically flows to love.

Then we can see and hear, taste, and smell, and touch Holiness, and feel it living and creating us. We sense constant beauty flowing as the river of life and we are baptized with water and blood flowing from the side of Christ.

It is obvious we are really stuck as a human race; we need help to see again. The Fall from Heaven was due to our capacity to be deceived, and the result is we are now deceiving ourselves, and others. Our darkness is deep, deeper than we can imagine. We are powerless to be free from our deception, or from being deceived. We have to face ourselves: this self-knowledge will arise when we strongly desire freedom from the ready-made reactions.

Our prayer that was so sweet now needs to become a wailing for help if we want to be free because now we see how deep our soul is drowning while trying to swim under its own power and getting farther from shore. Love is here to cradle us, yet she cannot lift us up if we stubbornly want to swim on our own, even if we are out of breath and dying.

What is handed down to us ancestrally is we are a 'child of fear, isolation, and ignorance and have been cast out of the Eden of Heaven.' Why? We are conditioned to 'have' knowledge rather than love. We continue to be power-crazy because ego is controlled by its desire to dominate the heart.

We are slaves. The spiritual chains of our personal prison are not known to us until it becomes too painful to bear any longer: we have to face our shadow that we cannot love without being at the center of that need. Even when love centers us, loves us, reconnects us, and creates us anew again, we still become distracted and 'run away' from love ..."

The above paraphrase is so direct and to the point that it may be a challenge to fully digest the powerful message and apply it to your life:

Let go of attachment to blood, the ancestral-genetic shadow we inherit from our parents.

Again, to participate with love and embody it fully, practice *Pratyahara*: orient inwardly, access your inner body space, and sense the sensations of the Divine therein.

Another way to take back our *Eros* - our will - so it belongs to us and then yield to love is to let go of our attachment to self-serving behavior patterns that are derived from the *Grail Wound*. The most direct way is to go straight inside and connect to *Eros*. Another way is to confront the strategies of the snake. Let's explore how the snake operates.

A DIVE INTO THE SNAKE

Like a parasite, the snake latches onto and uses our *Eros* to feed itself. When the snake drains our willpower, it perpetuates our false sense of a separate self, or ego, which creates more separation. Duality is the snake's dominion. One way to restore our will, or *Eros*, is to expose the snake's antics and make a snake confession to yourself, or another.

We are talking about rescuing our will, our *Eros*, from the snake that separates us from Divine Feminine Will. Do you find snakes' control of your *Eros* acceptable? If not, there is a way to shift what drives your *Eros* by owning your shadow.

Brene' Brown says, "Owning our story can be hard, but not nearly as difficult, filled with confusion, or suffering as spending our lives running from it. Embracing the vulnerabilities of our dark side is risky, but not nearly as dangerous as giving up on love, belonging, and joy - these are the experiences that open us to feeling vulnerable. Only when we are brave enough to explore, face, own, and feel the impact our darkness has on others will we discover the infinite power of our light." [42]

The following characterizations of the snake come from a profoundly personal, humbling journey into owning my shadow to face and feel the ways of my snake. My lessons are the result of reflections from a woman who lives the snake life fully. She once said to me, "I love living my snake life." How can someone love snake life? It is easy when the snake gets us whatever we want.

Before I consciously began my journey into the nature of the snake, I was strongly advised not to go there. Yet, I felt an inner knowing that "I HAVE to do this." Thankfully I had no idea how deep I needed to dive into the excruciating wormholes of my wound to face my core shadows and feelingly navigate them and survive the snake venom that I encountered. I was almost undone, to the horror of my support field of friends. Yet, by grace, I stuck it out despite the warnings that it would be my undoing. My snake journey was a series of initiations that made me stronger, more capable of self-love, self-compassion, self-forgiveness, and ultimately more capable of loving others.

In retrospect, it feels heartbreaking that some of us choose to live the snake life indefinitely, and remain imprisoned in an outer-directed, selfish life of *getting* from others. If so, we remain condemned by the delusion of false hope that something new outside of us - out there - is going to sweep us to freedom.

We seek a new relationship, move to another area to live, get a different job, buy new and better things, or start a project, etc. The reality is, without doing the painful inner work of owning our shadow, we will continue suffering the core feelings of *confusion of identity* - not knowing who we are, *feeling separate* and *alone* and *feeling incomplete* and *broken*. These deep core layers have no story. Whereas, there are also secondary stories such as fear of loss, self-doubt, and self-hatred due to a weak will. Meanwhile, the snake maintains control and tightens its grip on our *Eros*. Others not trapped by the snake's strategies see it clearly in us, yet, we cannot see the snake operating in ourselves, so we remain separate from love and unable to live life fully.

Instead, we live the snake life, and even profess to love it, and inevitably we also live a secret life. When alone, we suffer confusion, emptiness, despair, and loneliness. We lack a center, with no embodied grounding or safety, and we are without passion, other than to blindly achieve the snake's selfish agenda - even when it is against our will. It is devastating to realize how living a snake's life can be so overpowering an addiction. Yet the snake drains the will of our *Eros* until the enslavement becomes so compelling that we no longer have sufficient will to say 'no' to the snake. We remain unable to muster the will power to take the steps that open us to love and start to live a new lifestyle guided by love. Living imprisoned, with our will under the snake's control, ensures that we will not cross the threshold to freedom and unite with love. To break free, we have to turn inward, away from the snake, and reconnect to Divine Feminine Will, particularly if we desire to manifest our life's work.

HERMES' CADUCEUS, THE MIDLINE AND THE CHAKRAS

Recall Hermes' Caduceus, a winged vertical staff with two intertwined snakes coiled around it. The two snakes, *Ida* and *Pingala*, crossover at each of the seven chakra centers. When the two snakes functionally balance around the staff - which is the central channel called the *Sushumna* - there is bodily health, harmony, wholeness, and union with love. When the two snakes are in conflict, it creates an inner war between the masculine and feminine principles at each chakra center.

The right-sided snake is *Pingala*, which is the masculine-hori-zontal-head centered thinking that objectifies, sends our attention outward toward material things, and separates them by naming. Our will succumbs to the allure of the outer image and the influences of people and events. *Pingala* expresses the cranial wave. The left-sided snake, *Ida*, is the feminine-pelvic-sensual-vertical-body centered, inner sensing aspect that is guided by *Eros*, the wisdom of the body, which is a sensual pulse of love. The qualities of *Ida* correspond with the biodynamic tidal fields. *Sushumna* is the neutral column of stillness associated with the heart center.[43]

When we live under the control of the snake, we favor the masculine, brain, fear-driven separating principle. Then we objectify, attention goes outward, and *Pingala* takes over our will, and we fall into the hypermasculine disposition. Thinking controls our will by making all the decisions about what we 'do.' When we live in a hypermasculine disposition, it means our will is over-influenced by *Pingala*, the snake-brain. Again, operating from the snake-brain is a shadow expression of the *Kundalini*, the Sacred Force of Love. In the Bible, the snake-brain is the serpent, a decadent form of the *Kundalini* that provoked the fall of human consciousness, which banished Adam and Eve from the *Garden of Eden,* which marked the fall of human consciousness.

THE FALL OF HUMAN CONSCIOUSNESS

In his book *Requiem for Modern Politics,* William Ophuls characterizes the historical period when humanity began to suffer the body-mind split. He says that when the human brain neocortex exploded in size 8,000 years ago, the mind split from the body. This event, known as the fall, occurred when our center of consciousness 'fell' from the infinite heart center connecting all things into limited brain-centered thinking. The fall generated the narcissistic self-sense of ego that separated us from our body and disconnected us from a sensuous body-felt union with nature. As humans, we lost the conscious body-felt connection with all things. This neurological event occurred when the human race shifted from being hunter-gatherers to an agrarian life. One group of humans became adversarial to others to protect the land from the heathens. Adversarial life and ownership of property indicates that the snake-brain controls attention and will, directing it outward.

Brain-derived thinking emits gross, gravity-centered digital static and imposes a harsh pressure that smothers the guidance from our delicate heart field, crushing it as an organ of perception. The brain controls our action (will), which is our modern 'given.'

Prior to the fall, our attention flowed like a delicate breath between the heart field and nature as a sensuous body-felt perception that was free, united with love, and erotically connected with all things. Attention was inner-directed, heart-centered, vertical, embodied, and in an erotic union with nature and universal love, which is the creative principle of the Divine Feminine. The fall, therefore, implies a shift of our consciousness from the unlimited coherence of heart perception to a limited brain function that focuses on fulfilling the selfish needs of a separate me. In modern times, our organ of perception is the limited mind rather than the unlimited heart field that is in connection with The All. When attention is head-centered, the ego orients in a horizontal outer direction, which through thinking and naming separates us from *Eros*, each other, nature, and from the creative force of love.

Living in the head fosters the hypermasculine disposition by which *Pingala* takes over and controls our attention. The neurological power of mind directs our *Eros* outward and misuses our will for narcissistic gain. The snake is responsible for the fall of human consciousness, which banished humankind from a domain in which we enjoyed a body-felt unified heart consciousness that the Bible calls the *Garden of Eden*. Before the fall, the Serpent or *Kundalini* operated as the creative Sacred Sexual Force of Love in our 2nd chakra that unites all things. After the fall, the snake-brain separates all things, which are for my use.

> The snake is not a force we overcome by willing it away. Surrender to love is the only power that can free our attention and liberate our will.

As mentioned, the snake controls our will by objectification, and fixing attention outward onto objects, which recoils us away from an inner sensing of our *Eros* as the pulse of love. Ego imprisons our *Eros* by externalizing thinking. Rather than inwardly sensing as our organ of perception guided by heart-centered inner-body wisdom, our guidance is thinking that avoids fearful feelings and emotions based on our past.

SOCIAL MEDIA AND THE DESTRUCTION OF THE I

Rudolf Steiner wrote about the future decadent state of humanity nearly one hundred years ago, and we are on the threshold of what he predicted. In modern times, our seat of consciousness is drawn outward by the pulls of life, circumstances, and people. Social media is particularly concerning; its founders consciously instituted a proven highly addictive system based on B. F. Skinner's principles of behavioral modification. Hence, social media's methods of control ensure an addictive drive toward fulfilling our cravings. For example, we get a reward 'like' when we participate in social media, and the more 'likes' we earn, the greater it attracts virtual 'friends' who want to hear what our egos have to say. Our attraction to social media is not only addictive, it is also spirit crippling. It has the potential to destroy our flesh-to-flesh social fabric of interaction that can lead to an even deeper, unprecedented fall of human consciousness into a state of egoless non-individuality that is reflected by mass consciousness. Social media also reinforces the notion that somebody or something out there will rescue me.[44]

"Is it the snake, or love that drives my *Eros?*

"Who is driving the bus?"

DIFFICULTIES IN DIFFERENTIATING BETWEEN THE SNAKE AND EROS

We know only in retrospect that we have betrayed ourselves and followed the snake. For example, when we left a situation too soon that felt nourishing, or, we stayed too long, and we felt drained afterwards. Another form of self-betrayal occurs when we are with someone, and afterwards we feel empty, sad, unmet, and lonely, as opposed to feeling vitalized.

Fact is, if there is no erotic connection with a particular person, we will have nothing to do with them, and the same goes for places, events, or situations. *Eros* is the living substance that powers desire that, like glue, creates connection. *Eros*, when held inside without an object to project it upon, is guided by Divine Feminine desire that connects us with everything. What we do with our *Eros* or desire, is a direct bodily confession, like a physics equation: the more *Eros* we feel for someone, the more time we spend with that person, even if we are unaware of what controls our *Eros*.

> When we project our Erotic attraction, desire drives us to spend time with someone.

When the *Core Erotic Wound* controls our erotic attraction, desire is projected by ego toward someone to *get from* them for selfish gain, and we end up doing something that is against our authentic inner desire. We realize we have self-betrayed because we feel worse, afterwards. The question for self-inquiry is, 'what drives our *Eros*?' The snake's cleverness makes it challenging to differentiate between desire that is from snake and desire that is from an inner flow of love that longs for union with everything. To discern whether it is the snake or love that drives your *Eros*, ask yourself, "Is my desire projected out for selfish gain, or does my desire dwell within, while love softly guides my actions to serve for the good of the whole?"

Let's navigate the snake's recoil strategies to avoid the *Core Erotic Wound.*

7

OWNING YOUR GRAIL WOUND, PART 2

SNAKE TRACKS: HYPERMASCULINE, HYPERFEMININE, AND STILLNESS AS BYPASS

As mentioned, the snake symbolizes the brain and spinal cord that misuses thinking to collapse the heart field as an organ of perception to control your will. The snake becomes active when there is an overemphasis of the masculine head pole, the *Pingala*.

> When your will, which is erotic life force, is under masculine control, it radiates out to project an exalted self-image of *who you are not*.

Social media influencers, who have mastered the art of projecting an exalted self-image use deception to feed off of ordinary people. Their false appearance bodily confesses a misuse of the Luciferic qualities of beauty, awe, enamor, luxury and the lure of misguided *Eros* to manipulate others *to get* for selfish gain.

In the San Francisco Bay Area, where I lived for 40 years, there are hordes of 'gods' and 'goddesses' who dress up in their gorgeous costumes to shop in the hip organic stores and eat their vegan dishes at chic restaurants. Their Luciferic beauty projects a brilliant enlightenment that is too blinding for us ordinary folk to bear. Yet if we become enamored, we may try to emulate them.[45]

THE SNAKE WOUND IN THE HEAD CENTER: THE HYPERMASCULINE DISPOSITION

A person under the control of the snake looks beautiful, is head-centered, orients outward, and is focused on their appearance. One aspect of their projected over-exuberant false self-image is the pretense of being filled with lofty thoughts, brilliant ideas, profound realizations, and cosmic spiritual insights. Another sign that confesses living the snake life, is our websites are over the top beautiful and brilliant. A friend once lamented that she was frustrated and disappointed that no one responds to her website posting. I looked and thought, 'what a beautiful website,' but I also noticed that it was filed with unattainable aloof pontifications that did not represent who she is.

When together, two snake life driven people make plans about what's going to happen (future) due to their unique cosmic connection. However, their incredible schemes rarely material-ize. When the snake runs us, it is hard to concentrate, commit, follow-through, or even sit still because electrostatic charge creates an uncomfortable inner-buzz inside the body. A *Stillness Touch* session feels like torture when the snake is in charge because the stillness amplifies the sense of the inner war between *Ida* and *Pingala.* The conflict is between whether our desire is selfish and moved by fear or it is selfless and guided by love.

In contrast, without the snake in charge, a *Stillness Touch* session feels sensuously connected to *Eros*, which brings us closer to the *Self* and connected to others in the present. We feel reposed in the flesh of our pelvis, which feels sensuous, erotic, and in an inner-body contact with love.

THE SNAKE'S STRATEGIES OF RECOIL FRAGMENTS OUR CONSCIOUSNESS

The snake splits our consciousness into multiple fragmented parts. Each fragment displays narcissistic behaviors that are driven by specific psychological complexes, which fixates our attention on a particular dualistic adversarial perspective between an inside *me* versus an outside *you*. Therefore, awareness is outer-directed by the ego that objectifies a self-versus other. From this dualistic disposition, objectification is used to heighten the ego's false sense of separation, which intensifies the electrostatic qualities inside our body. The subsequent inner buzz makes it almost impossible to relax, unwind, be still, concentrate, be alone, or do nothing. As you read in an earlier paraphrase, because we are manipulating our attention all the time, we feel exhausted.

THE EGO MANIPULATES ATTENTION TO AVOID DISCOMFORT.

The snake, being narcissistic, possesses no witness consciousness for self-reflection. Therefore, when the snake is in control, we are not the owners of our attention or our will. Trapped in narcissism, we have no empathy and cannot feel the impact that our behavior has on others. Whenever we receive reflections from others about the uncomfortable impact our behavior has on them, we express genuine disbelief and then we deny, defend, argue, get angry, attack, and lash out. Such actions create more separation, which ego prefers, rather than to listen, digest, muster up the courage and humility to face ourselves, and with gratitude thank the other for helping us to see how we behave in ways that hurt people. Remember, when the ego is in charge, it refuses to recognize its antics.

Again, when the snake is in charge, our thinking, feeling-emotions, and will are based on the past or future. Emotionality drenches our stories, beliefs, memories, and will that determine our actions. Hence, we display volatile whipsaw behaviors that shift rapidly in opposite directions amid the slightest provocation. Therefore, sensitive people instinctively do not like us, and they are leery of our volatility. We innocently lament that we feel like an outsider and are lonely. Because our activities are selfishly oriented toward using others for self-gratification, people avoid us like the plague.

A DUALISTIC 'NON-DUALITY' THAT POSES AS ENLIGHTENMENT

The snake has an interesting way that it hijacks attention and projects it out as an exalted false self-image that looks like a classical awakening for others to see. Here, the snake confuses the natural laws of awakening and blurs natural boundaries by the misuse of language. Pontifications without realization abound, such as "it's all good," "everything is perfect just as it is," and "it is not spiritual if we do not love everyone."

Since the snake operates from a non-position of confusion of identity, we feel lost, separate, alone, bewildered, and without discernment, because we do not know ourselves, given that we have no contact with I AM. Without being connected to the midline of *Shivic* stillness as the positive masculine, we cannot discern who we are, what we stand for, what we can commit to, or who another is.

Nor can we differentiate between one type of cranial work from another, or one kind of tantra from another because "it's all one."

THE SNAKE HAS NO BOUNDARIES

The snake operates from a false *positionlessness* with no ability to take a stand because there is no center. Whatever happens with whomever - harmful or beneficial - is "perfect, because it is all love." "We love everything and everyone because we are all part of a global community." Meanwhile, displaying hypocrisy at its finest, we hide from ourselves and others our seething rage, hatred, jealousy, and resentment that we feel toward certain people, races, social classes, diets, or political situations. These are normal human reactions; it is the hiding them that makes us dangerous. Suppressing and hiding emotions are like loading a powder keg that is bound to blow up.

In contrast, authentic boundaries occur as inexplicable laws of nature that express bodily truths; we can discern that some folks are 'family' and others are not 'family' just like the slime mold does. Slime mold, the simplest life form on earth with no nervous system, possesses the discernment to avoid another slime mold by creating an impermeable barrier against it. Or, a slime mold will unite its body and become one with another slime mold.[46]

COMMITMENTS WITH NO FOLLOW-THROUGH

Another confusing action on behalf of a snake-driven person is with commitments. We quickly make plans that feed the ego's selfish needs, yet in contrast, we avoid anything that amplifies our inner-body presence of love. In a moment of grace, we may commit to a connection that generates love, and then we abort it as soon as a better option arises to get our snake's selfish needs fed. Recall that "we run away from love."

In our core essence we long to be united with love and intimately related to others. Even so, the snake hijacks our attention to control our will and weakens it to the point that we repeatedly do the opposite of what we know to be our core heart's desire. Therefore, we subsequently feel confused, powerless, guilty, ashamed, jealous, filled with anxiety, doubt, hatred, fear, a sense of loss, separation, isolation, and rigidity, all of which closes our heart field, and we feel like we are suffocating. Yet we keep on with 'The Work.' The core wound can drop deeper and infect the heart center.

THE NON-DUAL DISPOSITION AND THE HEART WOUND: STILLNESS AS BYPASS

A non-dual disposition can also indicate a wound in the heart center. Hordes of non-dual folks roam about in spiritual bypass by mis-using stillness to avoid reality. Zen Buddhists call it *stuck in emptiness*. This type of non-dualism is an abdication of an embodied realization of the heart's self-existing radiance as the center of the *Self*. Misusing stillness as bypass is prevalent among the more sophisticated intellectual seekers who have read the books and sat with the gurus. Such teachers instruct us to project a detached witness consciousness from the head center to peer down into the lowly body (that is not real). And this projection of attention into the body instead of submerging consciousness fully into the body is called embodiment.

When witnessing is poised from above, our consciousness is not submerged in the body, nor reposed in the self-existing heart radiance. Therefore, it is disembodied consciousness. Again, when witness consciousness is an objective observer that gazes down into an unreal body from a distance, it denies the body-felt heart union with our embodied sensuousness in the pelvis. When our presence disconnects from the sensuous qualities in our inner body, separation continues. Therefore, we remain dissociated and trapped in a subtle process of objectification and hatred of our dreaded body in the name of enlightenment. Witness consciousness exclusively oriented to stillness, and not united with the sensuous pulses in the body is a subtle hyper-masculine strategy that flourishes in non-dual circles. Admitting that we are stuck in emptiness may be too painful to own. Yet, as mentioned, we have to give up our spiritual accessories if we want to catch our ego and superego in the many strategic covert acts it employs to avoid reposing in the self-existing heart radiance and the sensuous intimacy of *Eros* in our body. It is a tricky navigation when we operate from a detached witness consciousness because it feels blissful, loving, and spiritual. Non-dual spiritual teachers are rampant in the San Francisco Bay Area, and they have infiltrated Europe, Australia, and Asia. Hordes of twenty and thirty years old 'realized masters' of non-duality market their brand of enlightenment and are getting rich off of innocent seekers. Their naïve perspective of non-duality denies the body, which is the quintessential creation of Divine Feminine Will that expresses love.

Stillness as bypass confesses terror of feminine power and hatred of the body.

I subscribed to this non-dual hatred of the body, nodding yes when my teacher said things like, 'I am not my body, I am not my thoughts, feelings, or actions. My body is a burden, a bag of garbage that I tolerate and drag around until the emptiness takes me out of it.' My friend, spiritual teacher Saniel Bonder, once heard a female guru declare, "I am not a woman!" when asked what is it like as a woman to be a guru?"

Advaita master Ramana Maharshi's comment below breaks my heart:

> "If true realization is attained, who wants this body? For a Realized Soul who enjoys limitless bliss through realization of the Self, why this burden of the body? A Realized Soul has really no love for his body. For one who is the embodiment of bliss, the body itself is a disease. He will await the time to be rid of the body. When he has the body, he has to clean its teeth, has to walk, bathe, and give food to the body, and has to do many other things besides. If a boil grows, it has to be washed and dressed; otherwise it becomes septic and emits a bad smell. In the same way, if the body is not kept clean, it will get diseased. A Realized Soul looks upon his body in the same way that a coolie regards his load. He will look forward to putting down the load at the destination." [47]

Perhaps the misuse of stillness as bypass is a necessary stage along the path of our evolution; yet at some point, we may have to decide if we want to evolve past the notion that only stillness is real, and choose also to include the sensuous embrace of Divine Feminine Love as an essential aspect of our nature.

Recall that the hypermasculine disposition collapses the heart field as an organ of perception, which eventually wears our will down to the point of utter exhaustion, which marks an even deeper collapse into the snake life: the hyperfeminine disposition.

THE HYPERFEMININE DISPOSITION AND PELVIC WOUNDING

The hyperfeminine disposition reflects a wound in the pelvis. It is marked by an exhausted, collapsed will, which is due to prolonged suffering under the incessant ravages of hypermasculine self-criticism, self-control, self-suppression, self-hatred, self-doubt, and self-fear. All the time we spend running from love and avoiding discomfort drains our *Eros* until our life force becomes so depleted that we lose grounding in the body, and veer from our center in the midline. In other words, by dissociating we lose contact with our essence.

DISSOCIATION

Once our will has been broken, we dissociate out of the body into the periphery of the outer cosmic domains of the runaway feminine energies. Runaway, in this context, implies being trapped in a domain that is so far out in the periphery it is without a center, with no anchor in the body. We are not embodied, we feel unsafe, nor do we have any connection to the ground of the earth. No contact with the body also means there is no connection to an embodied positive masculine principle as a core of stillness that provides us with discrimination, discernment, and boundaries. When the will collapses to this degree, we feel powerless and lost in the swirling peripheral hyperfeminine energies, which leaves an empty void inside us that fills our body with an inner buzz of subtle terror. We feel continuously irritated, paranoid, unsafe, confused, unable to be with adversity, and we avoid discomfort, intensity, intimacy, paradox, conflict, and confrontation. We have no strength of will to honor commitments, to discern or differentiate, to make decisions, take a stand, or to manifest our life's purpose.

There is no strength in our willpower, so we are under-resourced.

When our consciousness expands that far out into the peripheral feminine cosmic energies without a reference to the body, mother earth, or embodied positive masculine, and with no connection to our core midline of stillness, we become a helpless plaything, as we drown on the outer edges of the ever-changing swirls of the life currents that subject us to the whims of every shift. There is nothing to anchor us, which is necessary for integration. If we remain stuck in the collapse of the hyper-feminine disposition, we suffer immune system compromise, and an array of mysterious illnesses, pains, hypersensitivity, allergies, and diseases. This may lead to strict self-imposed dietary limitations, fasting, enemas, and other bodily depravations, which in the end can make us more ill. Our health comes crashing down, and we have not got the will to stop the downward spiral into a chronic disease.

If you are stuck in the hyperfeminine disposition, it is a profound wake up call, indicating that now is the time to begin your long, slow process of taking your *Eros* back so that it belongs to you. Your body is sounding the alarm: re-establish a deep relationship with your core midline of stillness from inside the flesh of your body, and reconnect with the inner positive masculine. If not, chronic long-term debilitating illnesses await you that resemble the fisher king who is condemned to his bed paralyzed and unable to rule the kingdom.

SUMMARY

The ego uses all the above strategies of recoil to avoid integrating the *Core Wound* due to hatred of the feminine and terror of her power. In review, the *Core Erotic Wound* impacts all three primary body centers head, heart, and pelvis. There is the narcissistic misuse of will by the head-centered hypermasculine, the nondual misuse of stillness as bypass in lieu of uniting with the heart radiance, and the paralysis of the will in the pelvic center due to the incessant hypermasculine ravages that lead to a collapse of the will into the hyperfeminine. These wounds in our three centers are expressions of the snake, which

128

prevent the realization of our spectral wholeness and deprive us of enjoying a sacred union between body, pure consciousness, and universal love as our fundamental birthright. However, there are also numerous secondary forms of recoil to navigate; so now let's explore the behavior of a man and a woman who is controlled by the snake. Please keep in mind that all this equally applies to both sexes.

THE SNAKE'S INFLUENCE ON MAN AND WOMAN: THE PLAYER AND MAN-EATER

A woman under the control of the snake is known as a man-eater, and the male equivalent is the player. A man-eater and player are usually physically beautiful and possess an irresistible charismatic sexual power that charms people who notice them in a crowd. Except for those rare ones who are awake, most men immediately fall in love with a man-eater, while awake women will instinctually despise her. The same applies to the players: gullible women will melt in his presence. Man-eater's and player's use their sexual prowess to covertly manipulate, seduce, and control the libido of their prey to get whatever they want from them for selfish gain, and then they throw them away when they are finished.

Famed protégée of Jung, Marie Louise Von Franz, wrote that a man cannot resist the power of a woman's *Eros* if she desires to have him. Von Franz hints that women have a moral responsibility that goes with the territory of having a female body that naturally expresses love. The same applies to the player: I know a man who confessed to me that in his peak years he would pick up three women a day at museums and public spaces and lured them to have sex with him.

When the snake manipulates *Eros* to get for selfish gain, it is a blatant misuse of power. In this case, it is a misuse of the *Sacred*

Force of Love, which is the power of *Kundalini*, the source of *Shakti* that dwells as *Eros* in the body. In his CD book, *Making Love*, Barry Long graphically characterizes the state of a woman whose *Eros* is under control of the snake. She uses her *cunt power* by dangling the possibility of sex to get whatever she wants from a man. As Long explains it, this occurs when a woman's uterus is so wounded and emotionally drenched that a psychological complex arises that controls her *Eros* 'to get' for selfish gain. Long says that the final expression of this complex is the *fiendess*. It is a man's most dreaded aspect of the negative feminine, and he will do anything to avoid it because the *fiendess* wields the threat of psychological castration, his greatest terror. The male equivalent of the fiendess is the enraged killer.

Snake Tracks Indicate an Unresolved *Core Erotic Wound*

A man-eater and player use prey to feed their insatiable sexual appetite for a myriad of reasons: to get orgasms, to relieve horniness, to release pent-up tension due to the emotional build-up of armor in the anus, prostate, penis, vagina, or uterus, to reduce anxiety, and decrease stress. But the snake also uses *Eros* to exploit men and women financially, to get housing, travel, fine dining, gifts, money, favors, coveted job positions, or other self-gain. Snake chews up and spits out its prey after using them for selfish gain: be it sexual, financial, social, psychological, or spiritual. Recall that the snake operates from the head center, co-opts our attention, and separates it from the love that pulses in the body. The snake fixates attention, moves it outward to objectify and separate itself from its victim to feed. The snake feeds off of other people's *Eros* like a parasite, which further empowers the snake and perpetuates the self-serving strategies of seducing, manipulating, teasing, withholding, controlling, throwing away, and then finding a new prey. Now let's characterize the snake tracks in the sexual domain. Again, this is not pretty.

CHARACTERISTICS OF SEX WHEN OPERATING FROM THE GRAIL WOUND

When we avoid our *Grail Wound,* it 'behaves' us by abusing our *Eros* to wield the snake's cunning. The snake misuses deceptive words, seductive body language, and emotional erotic magnetism to manipulate others' libido to get from them for personal gain.

However, *Eros* is our inner body connection to love, the power by which we achieve our life's purpose. In its mature form, *Eros* is our power to serve our unique gift that we offer as love to others and the world. When love pulses in our body, it generates more love in the world. An unintegrated *Core Erotic Wound* hinders our capacity to serve others because the wound is related to *Eros,* our generative, creative life force in the 2nd chakra, which is mostly unconscious. Therefore, it takes an act of the will to say no to the addictive pull of gravity due to the ego's self-centeredness, and free our attention to, instead, offer our *Eros* in the service of love. Otherwise, our *Eros* will remain a prisoner of the snake.

One indication that we suffer the effects of our *Grail Wound* is revealed by the quality of our sexual relations. When the *Grail Wound* drives our sex, it can be wild and animalistic, or cold and technique-driven. Both ways leave us feeling bereft, empty, sad, lonely, disappointed, and unmet after this kind of sex.

Another indicator that the snake controls our libido is addiction. In essence, we cannot stop having sex because our excessive animal need dictates that we repeat sex as often as possible during any given sexual encounter. Sex is not conscious, and the snake uses our partner's *Eros* to fill the bottomless pit of deficient emptiness that the *Core Erotic Wound* leaves in us. Bereft of the inner body wisdom of *Eros* to guide our sex, we objectify our partner and use them to feed off of by drinking their *Eros* to get local orgasms. Genital-centric orgasms temporarily relieve pent-up frustrations and dissipate our uncomfortable emotions and feelings, yet we suffer frustration and disappointment after snake sex. Anytime we use sex 'to get,' it is the snake. Long says both partners covertly participate in this unspoken collusion when they use one another to get orgasms. As mentioned, the snake is a psychological complex, a decadent personalized aspect of the Archetypal Serpent, the Sacred Sexual Force of Love, or the *Kundalini*.

> Every time we have snake sex it weakens our connection to love.

Misusing sex, withholding sex, teasing, and manipulating others libido to get something is how we avoid feeling the unbearable pain of our *Grail Wound*. The snake does not want us to be conscious and feel the impact of its antics because its control game would be over. Again, the snake is a powerful psychological complex that objectifies, fixes our attention and directs it outward to control our will. Snake is not interested in our cultivating the strength of will to do the painful work to recognize, face, own, feel, and unite with our *Core Erotic Wound*. Again, integrating our wound is the portal to union with love, yet we continue to misuse sex to manipulate and get from another, instead of communing body-to-body as Sacred Vessels of love.

> Having sex under the influence of the *Grail Wound* for selfish gain betrays what the Buddhists call 'right use of will.' It is crucial to understand that snake sex is not 'wrong' or 'bad.' We are learning how to love. However, to operate from our *Grail Wound* creates more suffering. Do we love living the snake life,

or do we let love guide us? Our bodily confession answers this question by what we do with our *Eros*.

As mentioned, *Eros* is our will, and love is the Divine Will. When we objectify our sexual partner and use them for selfish gain, it blocks our inner body connection with love. Without access to love as our guide, we do not receive inner-body cues that move our body that arise from the pulsations of *Pure Breath of Love,* and thus, we are cut off from the possibility of making Conscious Love.

When we love the snake more than love, then by default, we live by the dictates of the ego. Ego dwells in the thinking domain that is outside of our human design, it is the realm of inauthenticity - the *not-self* - and when operating from here we are disconnected from the flow of our *Tao,* the Divine Feminine Will. When our will disconnects from Divine Will, the Wisdom of the Whole, or *Prajnaparamita,* we feel separate, alone, and trapped in an empty hole of deficiency. We suffer fear, doubt, confusion of identity, self-hatred, guilt, inadequacy, jealousy, and shame. We also feel bereft of our birthright, which is a body-felt union with love. To avoid the discomfort of deficient emptiness, fear of loss, feeling broken, a confusion of identity, and aloneness due to a false sense of separation we abuse sex, drugs, social media, shopping, parties, food, or all of the above. This path of conditioning betrays our authenticity, innocence, joy, sensuality, and erotic freedom.

If living an authentic life interests you, instead of a conditioned one, the task is to face your *Core Erotic Wound,* which means to navigate it, integrate it, and unite with it.

THE CORE EROTIC WOUND AND OUR UNCONSCIOUS SOMATIC RECOILS FROM LOVE

Navigating our *Core Erotic Wound* means we make conscious all *unconscious* somatic and psychic recoils from love. We then consciously enter what Sri Aurobindo calls the core evil, which mirrors Christ's descent into hell that gave birth to his resurrection body.[48]

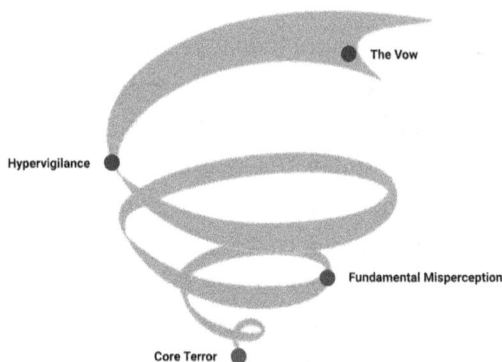

Figure 5. Navigation to Bring to Consciousness our Core Wound

As Figure 5 depicts above, the moment the *Core Erotic Wound* occurred, the ego took a solemn *vow* to never repeat it. Along with the vow, *hypervigilance* and a *fundamental misperception* arose, which led to the *core terror*.

The following navigation involves a bodily descent of your sensing presence into your flesh to bring to consciousness all aspects of your *Core Wound*. Let's descend into the depths of the body to unite consciousness with the *Core Erotic Wound*. This somatic navigation involves the following process:

- Cultivating a thorough understanding of your *Core Erotic Wound* (there may be more than one instance), and include your specific forms of physical, psychological, and practitioner recoil, and see them for what they are. Namely, recoils occur due to an unconscious somatic misperception of reality.

- Integration occurs by uniting your presence with your *Core Erotic Wound*, until gradually, you can be with all your recoils from love and they become conscious.
- A more grueling task is to remain present while navigating your unconscious choice points that have kept you from opening to love:

> *Discover your* Unconscious Vow,
> *Pinpoint your* Fundamental Misperception,
> *Articulate your* Subtle Core Terror.

Once you have integrated these uniquely personal insights, your spirit is free from ego's trap of narcissism (the snake) and you can evolve. Below is a suggested journey to help you discover your own somatic navigation as a *felt-sense inside your body*.

~

Your Somatic Journey into the Underworld

THE UNCONSCIOUS VOW

During your journey remember the *given*: the *Core Erotic Wound* is the most painful event in your life. The moment your *Core Wound* occurred, out of self-preservation the ego and superego took a solemn unconscious vow *(feel this somatically)*:

"Whatever it takes, I will never feel the pain of the *Core Erotic Wound*."

HYPERVIGILANCE AND THE FUNDAMENTAL MISPERCEPTION

The vow ignited a subsequent laser-sharp somatic hypervigilance to detect the slightest perfume-whiff of the *Core Erotic Wound*. Hypervigilance, in turn, generated the fundamental misperception. What is the Fundamental Misperception?

"Love is the *Core Wound*."

If the fundamental misperception spoke it may say (*feel this somatically*):

"If I let love flow freely within me, it will trigger the *Core Erotic Wound*."

THE CORE WOUND IS THE FULCRUM FOR OUR ARRESTED DEVELOPMENT

The *Core Wound* severed our body-felt connection with love, and remember, this event was so painful that it arrested our development. Therefore, we may remain developmentally stuck in the tender young place we were in the moment the core wound severed our body from love. From then on, the presence of love and the core wound became intertwined, which convinced us somatically that, "letting love freely express in my body will reactivate the *Core Wound*." As adults we know that letting love flow in the body will NOT reactivate the *Core Erotic Wound*; yet what drives our recoiling behavior is the unconscious misperception that *love is the core wound*.

Recall that the fundamental misperception is not verbal or intellectual; it is an *unconscious somatic misperception* therefore, self-talk and belief system modification will not remedy it.

Accompanying the fundamental misperception is a subtle core terror.

THE SUBTLE CORE TERROR

Right on the heels of the fundamental misperception there lurks the subtle core terror. If the *core terror* spoke, it might say *(feel this in your body):*

> "If I let love in, I will go crazy, I will be extinguished, it will kill me, ..."

Being aware of our hypervigilance, facing our fundamental misperception, combined with feeling our core terror creates an impossible paradoxical dilemma:

> "To become whole, I have to let love in, *and* it will kill me."

This is a dynamic tension of opposites choice point - a fulcrum that mirrors the Initiate journey into the depths of embodied self-development. Let's navigate it.

THE IDEAL JOURNEY WITHIN THE BODY

When we meditate, offer or receive *Stillness Touch,* or make Conscious Love, it builds the potency of *Eros. Eros* wells from the pelvis, moves up the midline into the belly, passes through the solar plexus to unite with the radiance of the heart to become a conscious emanation of love that suffuses love inside the whole body. This ideal journey occurs *if* we have <u>not</u> experienced the *Core Erotic Wound.* However, most of us received the *Core Erotic Wound,* our *given,* so here is our journey

OUR JOURNEY WHEN THE GIVEN IS PRESENT

Recall that after experiencing the *Core Erotic Wound*, the ego vowed to never repeat it, which requires hypervigilance to catch it. Therefore, upon the slightest whiff of a build-up of the potency of *Eros* hypervigilance activates unconscious physical recoils to stop love from moving up the midline.

FORMS OF RECOIL

Examples of physical recoil include, the cellular-level recoils from the gelled ground substance, defensive behavior patterns from the armor in the body, pelvic tension, gut tension, the knot of recoil in the solar plexus, the front and back heart knots, and throat tension. There are also the psycho-emotional recoils from the three primary body centers in the head (*doubt*), heart (*hatred*), and pelvis (*fear*).[49] Finally, during sessions, practitioners may engage recoils that impede *Pure Breath of Love*.[50]

All these recoils combined are the first line of defense designed to stop the flow of love. Again, always remember during your navigation, that these recoils are due to the fundamental misperception. Namely, the false belief that "the *Core Erotic Wound* will repeat if I let love rise from the pelvis into my heart radiance."

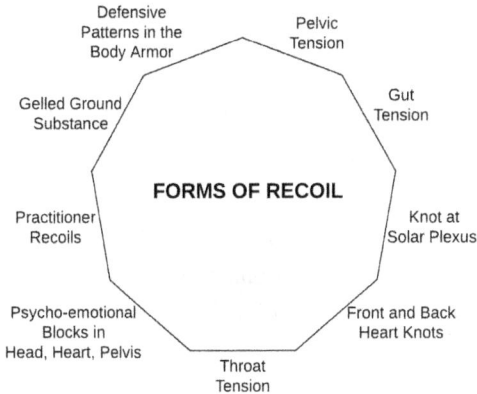

Figure 6. Summary of the Forms of Recoil Due to the
Core Somatic Terror

If, as a first line of defense, these recoils fail to stop *Eros* from rising to the heart radiance, then the superego unleashes the deep, hidden, core somatic terror that we have harbored in our flesh since the moment our initial *Core Erotic Wound* occurred.

Here are some examples of the Subtle Core Terror (bodily *feel them*):

If I let love in, the *Core Erotic Wound* will reactivate and

- I will not survive.
- I'll be alone forever.
- I will lose everything.
- I will die.
- I will lose myself in the infinite black abyss of nothing.
- I will no longer know who I am.
- It will destroy my life.
- It will extinguish my consciousness and I will no longer *be*.
- I will sit alone in a corner in a diaper, laconic, and drooling for the rest of my life.

- I will go insane.
- I will become an enraged killer, or an emotionally out of control fiendess.
- Everything I built up will come crashing down and life as I know it will end.

There are many variations of Core Terror, but they are not conscious, or verbal. Our extremely subtle somatic terror is wordless and lurks deep within the subconscious layers of our flesh.

All our life, the snake has misused our will, by wielding the dread of feeling our core terror as a weapon to control our attention and drive our will outward to abuse our libido to get from others. All to avoid feeling the pulse of love in our body in the name of never repeating the *Core Erotic Wound*. You can well imagine by now that the way to cross over the threshold to freedom is not easy, and it takes courage of heart.

CROSSING THE THRESHOLD

Crossing the abyss - from narcissism to freedom - is by a ferocious-hearted practice:

Dare to Face Your Core Wound and Feel Your Core Terror

CALL THE BLUFF

By analogy, this somatic practice is like being in a high stakes poker game between your embodied presence and the superego. The moment your *Eros* rises up the midline toward your heart radiance, the superego places a sure-fire bet that you will not dare to call. Here is an example of the superego's bluff:

"You will die if you feel love."

Yet, as a teacher during one of my meditation classes said,

"You have to gamble, call the bluff, and let love kill you."

If your calling the bluff is sincere, it makes conscious the entire charade of unconscious somatic, psychic, and practitioner recoils that were conjured up to avoid repeating the unbearable pain of the *Core Erotic Wound*. When all recoiling strategies become conscious, you are no longer at their mercy, and the subsequent integration leads to a union with the *Core Wound* that reveals a profoundly shocking realization:

BEING NOT SEPARATE FROM THE CORE EROTIC WOUND, YOU REALIZE PARADOXICAL CONSCIOUSNESS

Integration occurs after you are conscious of all aspects of recoil to love due to the *Core Wound;* that means you have united your presence with the wound, which, paradoxically, makes you whole.[51]

I am aware that sharing this practice is irresponsible if I were speaking to the general public. But you are in a practice to serve others, which requires that you have done your inner work, and you have cultivated the psychological stability to engage the practices.[52]

After reviewing a summary of the entire *Core Erotic Wound* navigation in Figure 7, let's explore specific aspects of *Stillness Touch*.

THE CORE EROTIC WOUND AND OUR UNCONSCIOUS
SOMATIC RECOILS FROM LOVE

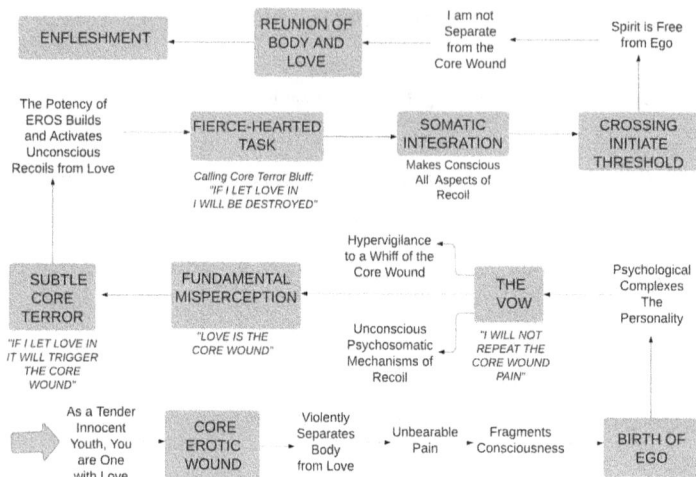

ENFLESHMENT ← REUNION OF BODY AND LOVE

I am not Separate from the Core Wound ←

Spirit is Free from Ego

The Potency of EROS Builds and Activates Unconscious Recoils from Love

FIERCE-HEARTED TASK → SOMATIC INTEGRATION

Calling Core Terror Bluff:
"IF I LET LOVE IN
I WILL BE DESTROYED"

Makes Conscious All Aspects of Recoil

CROSSING INITIATE THRESHOLD

Hypervigilance to a Whiff of the Core Wound ←

SUBTLE CORE TERROR ← FUNDAMENTAL MISPERCEPTION ←

THE VOW ←

Psychological Complexes The Personality

"IF I LET LOVE IN
IT WILL TRIGGER
THE CORE
WOUND"

"LOVE IS THE
CORE WOUND"

Unconscious Psychosomatic Mechanisms of Recoil

"I WILL NOT
REPEAT THE
CORE WOUND
PAIN"

As a Tender Innocent Youth, You are One with Love

CORE EROTIC WOUND

Violently Separates Body from Love → Unbearable Pain → Fragments Consciousness →

BIRTH OF EGO

8

STILLNESS TOUCH: A POST-BIODYNAMIC PRACTICE

W hen you give or receive a *Stillness Touch* session, your practice is to rest your attention *within* your body while your presence savors the subtle nuances of sensations that arise. It may be challenging to be with your inner sensuous qualities because they are paradoxical when you are in contact with stillness. Prolonged contact with Dynamic Stillness facilitates its implosion into your inner body space, which becomes infinite and unites body, consciousness, and love. By reposing in this *inner body infinity*, you enjoy radiant consciousness, enhanced capacities of trust, indestructible innocence, receptivity, and safety amid an open, undefended heart. Your increased strength of will enables you to remain present amid extremely uncomfortable emotional intensity and profound intimacy while your flesh trembles amid the pulsing of *Pure Breath of Love*. You easily repose in what arises without being controlled by the ego's strategies that recoil us from love.

If you continue your daily inner meditative practice, your thoughts, emotions, speech, body, and actions become free from the dizzying array of efferent, separating strategies of recoil on behalf of the limiting, controlling, narcissistic ego. You can remain present during activated traumas that are triggered by the release of the armor in your flesh, while your body expresses intense somatic recoil, painful memories, emotions, or re-enacts of uncomfortable old relationship patterns.

The ego avoids discomfort because it is too intense for it to bear, so it employs a multitude of strategies in an attempt to recoil your awareness to avoid feeling it, which as we now know, effectively cuts off love, as well as impedes the evolution of your consciousness. Abiding *inwardly* in stillness with free attention, while being present to sense uncomfortable intensity transmutes intensity into stillness. Then infinite stillness implodes within and emanates *Pure Breath of Love* as a uniting substance that harmonizes all polar aspects, which become expressions of love. When love suffuses your flesh, it frees your awareness, softens body armor, and unites your thoughts, speech, body, and consciousness until you can surrender to love that pulses in your body and connects you with all that is.

The Wisdom of the Whole, is known as *Prajnaparamita.*

YOU REALIZE YOUR BODY IS CONSCIOUSNESS SUFFUSED WITH LOVE

As mentioned, *Stillness Touch* is a gateway to an embodied inner union between pure consciousness and universal love that we call enfleshment. By its practice, you realize an utter non-separation *in your body*. If that interests you, it behooves you to cultivate a daily practice of sitting in stillness while you gain experience offering and receiving *Stillness Touch*. Again, your disposition is the same whether it is *Stillness Practice*, or *Stillness Touch*: inwardly orient your attention to be with what arises, *sense* it *as it is*, while you touch in non-doing and not knowing.

You do not need to mentally contrive a relational field of empathy, create a pseudo safe space for containment, make up the existence of a zone, or visualize virtual primary respiration. Neutral touch inherently creates all that is required for safety and embodied grounding that precisely matches what the recipient needs. Non-doing repose in innocence while touching also cultivates authentic boundaries that are inherent to embodiment, containment, and centering for the recipient. This provides a protection field for anything that arises, be it emotional intensity, intimacy, paradox, desire, transference, countertransference, or projection. When you are not efferent, *Pure Breath of Love* is free to evolve you and the recipient in the exact way needed in each moment.

Pure Breath of Love does not need a practitioner to help her out.

Your neutral touch synchronizes with and inherently matches the tempo of primary respiration that breathes in a recipient's subtle body. This tonal match arises naturally by the laws of entrainment *if* you can neutrally touch. To touch your recipient in neutral means that you orient *inwardly* to sense the inner body sensations in you, while you repose in non-doing and not knowing with no agenda or a goal. Then, you instinctively synchronize with the potent forces of primary respiration that well and recede within you *and* the recipient. While touching, remain mindful to keep your attention oriented *inward* while you sense the qualities *inside your body*. That is the fundamental practice for building the required strength of presence to open and yield to the spectral wholeness that unfolds within the potency of *Pure Breath of Love*. Cultivating a stable inner presence is a crucial protection field and container for all that arises.

Remaining present to the qualities of your inner sensations amid any degree of intensity, intimacy, or paradox, cultivates the courage of heart and the *strength of will* to not fall into the temptation of objectifying your recipient by projecting your awareness into their body to evaluate the anatomical parts to fix or heal them. Instead, you trust the tide in its unerring potency to reestablish wholeness in the recipient.

Whatever arises during your neutral touch, always practice the fundamental disposition:

> Let it be, leave it as it is, let go in open hearted repose, amid 'don't know.'

PREPARE YOUR RECIPIENT BEFORE TOUCHING THEM

While offering *Stillness Touch,* an emotional intensity may arise that is stored in the recipient's skin. Recall that skin is ectoderm, an embryological tissue layer that defends and protects us. Besides the skin, ectoderm also becomes the nervous, hormonal, and immune systems that are responsible for the self-recognition system and the stress fight-flight response. Emotions stored in skin arise from past hidden transgressions of our boundaries, so it may be challenging for a recipient to be with the discomfort of emotional intensity or shock that releases from the flesh during *Stillness Touch.*

Therefore, *before* the session begins, encourage your recipient to orient awareness *inwardly* to sense the qualities as they arise. You can tell them, "when you orient your attention inward, it creates a protective container that gives you the strength of presence to be with what arises *as it is.*" You can mutually share your experiences of the session *afterward*, encouraging the recipient to speak unedited.

> Do not tell your recipient what you 'think' they are experiencing.

DO NOT TALK DURING A SESSION: BE STILL

Unlike functional treatments, during *Stillness Touch* you do not talk *during a session*, and you do not verbally negotiate hand contacts. Nor do you name events or tell the recipient what you think is happening. Also, there are no treatment protocols in a *Stillness Touch* session. Nothing is pre-planned or goal oriented. Also, when you offer *Stillness Touch*, you do not orient to the nervous system, to anatomy, or to the cranial wave. In fact, you do not expect any motions to arise, even primary respiration, the tides, or *Pure Breath of Love*. Also, harbor no intentions, do not suggest stillpoints or visualize tides, attempt to relieve symptoms or treat: 'be still.'

> Stillness Touch is mapless with no expectations of any motions. Your touch is instinctually offered in conscious unknowing and non-doing.

YOUR INNER PREPARATION

Before you touch, pre-arrange signals with your recipient that indicate 'yes' or 'no' so that any time a recipient is struggling to *be with* the discomfort of intensity, intimacy, or paradox, he or she can signal 'yes' or 'no' to indicate whether they feel able to be with what's here, or not.

Once the recipient is comfortable on the table, begin your preparation: you orient *inwardly*, abide inside your heart space toward the spine, while whole-body breathing into your pelvic floor, which grounds your presence *in your body*. Meanwhile, sense the qualities of buoyancy arising in your inner body space. Once you have landed *inside* your body and you feel reposed in non-doing and not knowing, you can touch your recipient's body in the way that the *wisdom in **your** body* guides you, which is already in entrainment with the recipient's inner body wisdom.

Start your *Stillness Touch* at a place on the body where your *innerness* guides you, and stay there until you feel *inwardly* moved to touch somewhere else on your recipient's body. The depth of your touch, its quality, the tempo of your bodily movements, and the number of places you touch, arise from the guidance of the tones that you sense *inside **your*** inner body space: nothing is prescribed.

> Let the wisdom of your body guide your touch. Regard each hand contact as a fulcrum of stillness with no agenda. Every place you touch on your recipient is also a fulcrum of stillness that reflects the wisdom that emanates from your radiant heart field.

As mentioned, when you orient your attention inwardly, it invokes the laws of entrainment, and then your hands move by a hidden inner guidance from the *wisdom of the body*. Guidance arises from neutral touch that connects your inner body wisdom with the wisdom in your recipient's body. Your hands instinctively rest in stillness while you touch your recipient with reverence and awe as though their body is a sacred expression of love. Again, your hand contacts derive life, motion, gesture, and guidance to the places to touch by inwardly attuning to the tonal nuances of the sensations in ***your*** inner body.

PRACTITIONER DISCRETION THE FIRST TIME RECEIVING STILLNESS TOUCH

It is not a rule, yet sometimes you will sense that a recipient who is new to touch harbors anxiety. They may need more time to acclimate to the increased intensity, intimacy, and paradox that *Stillness Touch* evokes, particularly the first time receiving it. Let the recipient know at the beginning of the session *before you touch* all the areas that you might touch. Point to those places on your body and say, "during the session I may be touching your sacrum, belly, pelvis, chest, neck, jaw, thighs, calves, feet, etc., are you comfortable with that?" Wait for permission from the recipient, and watch for the secondary signals in their body language that mean 'no' despite having said 'yes.'

Silently honor the wisdom of the recipient's body. When their body language indicates 'no,' do not touch that area during the session. Sometimes we will say 'yes' while the body indicates 'no' and other times, a verbal 'no' is a bodily 'yes.' Also, if the recipient seems anxious or vigilant about being touched, start your touch in the periphery, and gradually move to the center. For example, start at the feet, and after you sense that the recipient has relaxed, then you can go intuitive and gradually move to areas closer to the core midline.

AUTHENTIC BOUNDARIES

Cultivating your discernment and sensing your recipient's *authentic boundaries* is a delicate navigation; it is a crucial skill when you offer *Stillness Touch* for the evolution of consciousness. This is an opportunity for you to attune inwardly, synchronize with what's here, and by entrainment to resonate with a recipient's authentic boundaries that lie beneath their ego-driven ones that are based on fear of repeating a core wound trauma from the past. Your refined attunement tonally matches your recipient's bodily wisdom; this cultivates trust that your recipient has in you so she can openly receive your touch while surrendering her body to love. The fruit of a practitioner's neutral is expressed as a non-contrived repose inside your body; you wait amid non-doing and not knowing while synchronized with the *wisdom of your body*.

Once permission to touch your recipient is obvious, abide *inside* your inner body space and attend to your sensations with presence, and then touch the places where you are inwardly guided. You repose in not knowing amid non-doing; this is a disposition of innocence while you orient inward with free attention, which allows your recipient's chakras, meridians, Bindu points, and central channel to spontaneously open to the infinite potency of the *Pure Breath of Love*. You may notice a whole-body pulse in your recipient and in yourself that is synchronized with the heartbeat and it is everywhere you touch. This pulse is *Spanda* or *Pure Breath of Love*. When *Pure Breath of Love* arises, you are free to touch the areas of the body that are rich with lymphatics.

STILLNESS TOUCH TO THE LYMPHATICS IS A GATEWAY FOR DEEP TRANSMUTATION

Once you sense the *Sacred Pulse of the Spanda* body-wide, *and* you feel inwardly guided to do so, touch the areas of the body that are rich with lymphatic vessels. For locations of the lymphatics, refer to an anatomy atlas such as Netter. *Stillness Touch,* when applied to the lymphatics in the presence of a whole-body *Sacred Pulse*, is a specific gateway that reveals to a recipient how they have habitually regarded their sensuousness in the past. Be aware that a recipient may welcome or shun revelations from the inner feminine wisdom that are evoked by the whole-body pulse of love, as we will explain.

Before you begin Stillness Touch to the lymphatic fields, you may, at your discretion, inform your recipient that unsavory personality traits may present themselves while you touch. This prepares a recipient to bear the difficult aspects of shadow that arise from the *Core Erotic Wound*, so let them know ahead of time that it may be challenging to *receive* the uncomfortable revelations about their history. Let your recipient know that all revealed information helps them realize their spectral whole-ness. Encourage your recipient to *be with* the given aspects of revealed history that formed the personality. You can suggest to your recipient that, "being with all of what you are is an aspect of *knowing thyself.* When you can welcome all of yourself with unconditional presence, it prevents self-critical judgment, shame, self-hatred, guilt, or labeling any self-discovery as bad, wrong, or evil. Whatever arises, let it be here *as it is* with an open heart."

> *Pure Breath of Love* can support a recipient during this whole-making process *only if* the practitioner is neutral and a recipient receives by letting in whatever arises.

When you are inwardly guided to do so, touch areas that are richly laden with lymphatics such as the jaw, neck, upper back, and under the arms. Again, touching the lymphatics will likely illuminate the deep core wound emotional history that is stored here. Opened lymphatic portals release trapped emotions that reveal to us the ways we have cruelly regarded and mistreated our body's primal *Eros* in the past. Lymphatics are an expression of chakra two, which is the fulcrum for the expression of the *Shakti,* which is the divine feminine principle in our body. Chakra two is in the sacrum, the Sacred Bone, that houses the *Kundalini,* the Sacred Force of Love, which is the power of our sensual desire for creativity, connection, and beauty in our lives.

One more suggestion, at your discretion, if you feel the recip-ient is mature enough to hear it, say to them, "while you are receiving lymphatic touch, you may feel the impact that self-criticism, self-hatred, or cruel treatment of your body has had on you and your beloveds. Yet by being with it you gain vital insight into how this has hindered the realization of your life's purpose. All you do if that arises is *let it be.*

When you are present with what arises *as it is*, intensity self-resolves into stillness.

You are prepared, as is your recipient, and you can begin touching the peripheral lymphatic areas of the body. When you have completed your touch to the peripheral lymphatic zones, you can touch the core erotic midline lymphatic fields in the throat, chest, solar plexus, belly, lower pelvis, perineum, and groin. Remain mindful that you continuously access stillness and repose in your pelvic breathing portal, which slows down the inner tempo of the thinking mind, which provides grounding while you touch these core midline emotion-laden areas. Remember, do not enter their subtle body field to sense inside the recipient; stay inside yourself. The depth and quality of your touch is derived from the inner body guidance derived from the qualities of sensation *inside you*.

> When in neutral inner attunement, the wisdom of your body will silently communicate with the bodily wisdom inside your recipient, which guides your touch. Neutral touch is crucial so you do not enter your recipient's inner space. Repose in your inner body and leave *Pure Breath of Love* in charge.

When you are in contact with the stillness inside you, your recipient can relax into the arising *innate bliss*, which is an illuminative substance *inside their body* that strengthens their ability to remain present to what arises amid the intensity, intimacy, and paradox. Continue your *Stillness Touch* to each area, and recall that anytime the whole-body *Sacred Pulse of the Spanda* is present, love moves your hands.

> *Spanda* is *Pure Breath of Love,* the most potent power on earth.

Spanda emanates infinitely and infinitesimally throughout the recipient's whole inner body, while suffusing love into the ground substance and within every cell. *Spanda* pulses in tandem with the heartbeat that is initiated by the sinoatrial node as the presence of love that suffuses every cell throughout the whole body.

Amid *Pure Breath of Love*'s whole-body pulse, you can trust that the session is in the hands of *Primordial Mother Love*, which takes into account the good of the whole. When you are neutral, the pulse of *Pure Breath of Love* is sensed by the recipient while it pulses inside you at the same time.

> The Sacred Pulse transmutes all that arises into *Pure Breath of Love*.

When touching your recipient, always inhabit your inner body space while you sense the tonal qualities therein. Your practice of maintaining *innerness* transmits love, by entrainment, to your recipient, along with the necessary containment, safety, trust, centering, and embodied grounding they need so they can receive the self-knowledge and inner guidance that arises from *Pure Breath of Love*. A recipient can repose in the trust that *inner body wisdom* guides you, which expresses micro-nuances of inner body tone moment by moment.

When you let your inner sensations guide the depth and quality of your touch, it is neutral, entrained, and in a precise tonal match with the tonal qualities emanating from the recipient's inner body wisdom. *Pratyahara*, which is orienting your aware-ness *inward*, replaces your previous habit of using efferent treat-ment skills that are driven by ego's need to objectify your recipient based on the notion of fixing or healing them. Instead, the quiet inner body pulse of love moves your hands, while you repose in the 'don't know' of *Divine Ignorance*.

You touch in silence while synchronized with the sensuous wisdom in your inner body space, which frees your recipient's will, strengthening it, so that he or she can be with any intensity, intimacy, and paradox that arises. The recipient can bodily repose within and trust amid the whole-making process and enjoy it without fear of being dis-empowered. An ambitious practitioner will tell you what they 'think' is happening inside you, or they may push you toward a goal, goad you into overwhelm, or manipulate the anatomy by efferent methods until the biodynamic field of primary respiration collapses into nervous system motion that expresses false fulcra as cranial wave motion patterns.

> The presence of the cranial wave is a sure-fire way to tell if you are efferent.

If you touch without objectification, in silence, amid non-doing and not-knowing, it ignites the laws of entrainment, and a recipient will feel as though your touch is arising from the wisdom within them, rather than from someone 'out there.'

To repeat, when in neutral, without objectification or efference, your touch is non-separating, which engenders in your recipient such a deep trust in you that she can repose in receptivity while *Pure Breath of Love* engages the process of whole making. Uncomfortable intensity will likely arise, remember that your prearranged signals are so your recipient can indicate 'yes' or 'no.' When your recipient is struggling to *be with* the discomfort of intensity, intimacy, or paradox, they can signal 'yes' or 'no' to indicate if they feel able to be with what's here, or not.

As a reminder, if the recipient indicates 'no' meaning, 'I cannot be with this right now' gently remove your contact and sit for a moment quietly to give your recipient time to acclimate to the intensity. Then move your hands to the next fulcrum you are guided to and touch it.

If the signal is 'yes,' indicating, 'I can be with the intensity,' you may, at your discretion, remind your recipient to practice sensing inside their inner body space, even if it feels intense, intimate, or paradoxical. The practice of *inner sensing* strengthens your recipient's embodied presence, and they will feel safe amid ever-deepening intensity. Your recipient can repose in implicit trust in the wisdom of their body until they feel the confidence to surrender to love. You mutually cultivate confidence together, which empowers you both *to be with* any intensity, intimacy, and paradox until you gain the strength of will and the presence, to *be with* whatever arises and leave it as it is.

Therefore, you and the recipient mutually cultivate inner sensing presence that engenders the safety, trust, receptivity, embodied grounding and strength of will to access *authentic boundaries* amid intensity, intimacy, and paradox without any sense of urgency, feeling rushed to a goal, or being efferently shoved into the cranial wave.

> Your practice is: *Wait, be still, and know that love is in charge.* Love prepares you to face your most deep-seated core wound issues.

RECOILS MAY ARISE DURING TOUCH DUE TO THE CORE EROTIC WOUND

We have covered many aspects of recoil due to the *Core Erotic Wound,* and they are likely to arise during your touch. You may recall that once *innate bliss* is freed, it reveals how you have habitually treated your body and its sensuousness. *Innate bliss* exposes the disposition you had toward your body, the feminine principle, your sexuality, and the sacred force of love, the

Kundalini, that is inherent to chakra two. Since you are also touching the skin, remember that the skin stores, and thus can reveal painful memories that have evoked the unconscious neurological recoil at the solar plexus. Touching the skin may initiate ego's clinging and recoil patterns that are held in the ectoderm. Again, the ectoderm is the embryological layer of defense that develops into the skin, immune, hormone, and nervous system that stores the prior transgressions of your boundaries by others, or through self-betrayal. *Innate bliss* that arises during *Stillness Touch* gently reveals the stored aspects of a recipient's history and resolves them, so all we do is repose in presence.

Always base the guidance of your neutral touch on the quality of the *presence of stillness* inside you, which ensures that the tempo of your touch is slow enough so that a recipient can *be with* the intense emotions and memories and will be able to digest the insights that arise, which cultivates sufficient trust and grounding in *presence* to remain receptive to the process. The recipient can confidently navigate their personal shadow issues that are stored as emotion-laden armor in the body, moment by moment, as the *innate bliss* gently reveals them. Amid profound intensity, recall that each issue that we face with presence transmutes to love. Likewise, when a recipient is present amid each aspect of their shadow, one by one, like a portal, it opens their whole body to love. The mutual cultivation of a stable presence prepares both recipient and practitioner for being present to the deep *Core Erotic Wound* issues when they arise.

> The *Core Erotic Wound* recoils are the result of traumatic events that severed our bodily connection with our Eros at a tender age.

The excruciating core wound created the deep personality traits of recoil that we struggle with for the rest of our lives. After receiving a sufficient number of sessions that the recipient needs to cultivate and enjoy unwavering presence, safety, implicit trust, grounding, and the cultivation of authentic boundaries, *Stillness Touch* to the lymphatics will run its course.

As an aside, this does not imply that you offer lymphatic sessions per se, you touch the lymphatic areas *only* when you are guided to do so while you are neutral.

REVIEW OF YOUR PRACTICE WHILE OFFERING STILLNESS TOUCH

To repeat, your practice when you offer *Stillness Touch* to the lymphatics or anywhere else on the body, is to orient your attention inwardly, while attuning to the sensations in your inner body, and let your sense of the tone in the qualities *inside you* be in charge of all aspects of your hand contact. Namely, the pressure, depth, and how your hands move on and off the body, where you touch, how you move about in the room, even picking up of your chair are all guided by the potency of your inner body wisdom.

A key to transmission in any domain in life, be it *Stillness Touch*, meditation, teaching, making love, or while in the market-place, is to remain inwardly connected to the qualities inside you. It is the innerness that inspires love to suffuse your thinking, feelings, and will (head, heart, pelvis). Your touch will feel 'right' to a recipient when you are entrained with their flesh by attuning to *your inner body* qualities. Your recipient can surrender to your touch because she can sense that your guidance arises from the wisdom within *you* that is also in entrainment with her body's inner wisdom.

To offer neutral touch that feels 'right' to a recipient, it is crucial that you do *not* let your attention efferently leave your body, pass through your hands and enter your recipient's subtle body to evaluate them, feel for cranial wave imbalances, or orient to the nervous system and anatomy to relieve symptoms, heal, or find wholeness. Instead, keep awareness inside you at all times. That leaves *Pure Breath of Love* free to illuminate memories, emotions, static, electricity, armor, shock, trauma, and any aspect of recoil due to the *Core Erotic Wound* that is stored in your recipient's flesh, which when suffused by stillness, amid presence, transmutes into love. In neutral, a practitioner is not doing anything except repose in, *'be still and know I AM.'*

A RECIPIENT'S PRACTICE: INTENSITY, INTIMACY, PARADOX ARE PORTALS TO LOVE

Once a recipient receives several *Stillness Touch* sessions, they will learn to effortlessly attune to the sensations within the body and let love be in charge, which guides their boundaries, choices, and the degree of intensity, intimacy or paradox they are willing to face and feel. Again, it is an inner *body wisdom* that by entrainment directs your hands to touch places with the precise quality and depth that matches what your recipient needs. This cultivates in your recipient an implicit trust in the process, regardless of the intensity, intimacy or paradox that arises.

> Remember this occurs by reposing inside you, not by entering the recipient's body.

DISTINGUISHING BETWEEN INTENSITY, INTIMACY, AND PARADOX

Intensity refers to emotionality that unconsciously drives the reactivity of recoil from love due to fear of repeating your painful history. Whereas intimacy is the relationship you have with aspects of *Self* and reflects your capacity to be with what arises, and whether you can let love flow freely in your body. Paradox arises after letting love in, which facilitates the union between body, consciousness, and love. When your physical and spiritual essences unite, opposing qualities co-exist in a baffling harmony.

WHAT IS INDESTRUCTIBLE INNOCENCE?

Amid all three gateways of intensity, intimacy, and paradox, regardless of what arises your practice of innocence, as stated earlier, remains the same:

> Let it be, leave it as it is, and let go into an open-hearted repose amid 'don't know.'

Each inner body quality emanates a specific tone that is a gateway for cultivating the presence to be with what arises, be it thoughts, feelings, emotions, memories, expanded spiritual states, etc. You cultivate this capacity to be with all that arises during a *Stillness Touch* session and by your daily stillness meditation practice. Once your practice of *being with what is*, and *leaving it as it is*, bears fruit, it becomes your core of *indestructible innocence*.

This primordial innocence is your original protection field that existed prior to any wounding. In due course, through the practice of being with your inner body sensations, you enjoy a continuous, unbroken contact with the love that creates all that is. This inner body union becomes so deep that there is no discernable difference between the primordial tender mother love and your flesh because they have become one.

> An all-cell, bodily union with *Pure Breath of Love* is enfleshment. When love moves, your body moves and erotically connects with everything.

The practice of inwardly *being with* cultivates the strength of will for you to enjoy the unflinching presence to *be with* ever-increasing intensity, intimacy, and paradox.

All the lifelong strategies that ego misused to recoil love and block the union of body, consciousness, and love will arise for your recognition. *Being present with* what is and not wavering into avoidance or over-enamor transmutes everything into love.

> Love is the unrestricted flow of life force in your body.

As each gateway of recoil opens in your body, it liberates the pent-up life force that creates the knots of recoil in your subtle and physical body. Life force is *Eros, Shakti, Prana, Spanda,* the *wisdom of the body, innate bliss,* or *chi* that when free illuminates all the blocked areas in the subtle body that create body armor, revealing associated emotions that are related to your history. If you can be with what arises, it strengthens your presence to be with increasing degrees of intensity, intimacy, and paradox. Amid this gradual increase of the strength of your will, you cultivate the *presence of stillness* to *be with* any arising, no matter how challenging.

> *Presence of Stillness,* as a strength of will, is the door to a *Completion Stage* realization.

You gain self-knowledge about aspects of your *given* history that unconsciously limits you. These are your hidden personality quirks and habits that are from your conditioning that prevent you from opening to love, and which hold you back from fully living your authentic life. You can live your authentic life by a continuous realization of a union between body and love. While you enjoy continuous contact with love, it guides you to your authentic boundaries, by which you realize your life's purpose.

Opening with presence to a specific issue as it arises is a way that each bodily gate becomes a portal for navigating your personal 'map' that shows you exactly how your ego's strategies have blocked you from love. *Being with* each of your blocks, and the correlating behavioral issues that connect to it, teaches you how to be with all the strategies of ego that recoil, cling, dissociate, control, hold back, or collapse amid intensity, intimacy, and paradox due to powerful surges of *Spanda* pulsing as love.

Again, whether you sit daily in stillness, or receive and give *Stillness Touch*, your practice is to sense inwardly and be with any degree of intensity, intimacy, and paradox that arises. Your challenge is to remain present amid all of ego's recoil from love: be it as thoughts, emotions, feelings, memories, or physical recoils at the solar plexus. Neutral touch brings all of these into your awareness gently, so you are not engulfed or overwhelmed by the paradoxical interface between self-limiting personal love and the boundless power of universal love.

Exploring the bodily gateways of touch is grounded in stillness so that you can segue from one level to deeper levels at a slow, gentle pace. While you repose in an unwavering presence amid ever-increasing intensity, intimacy, and paradox, the quality of your touch deepens as the spiritual depth increases, and this creates a holding space for all that arises.

A HOLDING SPACE IS THE BOUNDARY FOR FREEDOM

A holding space is a protection field for containment that is mutually created between you and your recipient while you offer neutral touch. During touch, both participants drop inside stillness while whole-body breathing to inhabit the inner body space to *be with* and sense the qualities of sensations; this provides centered, embodied grounding.

An advanced practice, while you orient inward, is to rest in the inner breathing portal at the back of your heart while you repose in the breathing portal of your pelvic floor that is connected with the core heart of mother earth. This practice combines your heart radiance with the sensuousness of *Eros* that unites with the core heart of mother earth, and the Divine Feminine Will.

> A holding space is a mutually created inner body atmosphere sealed in stillness and under love's protection that allows everything *to be*.

Allow and let be the entire spectrum of being and all its possibilities. Include your sensations, thoughts, feelings, emotions, moods, memories, somatic experiences, bodily recoil at the solar plexus, body movements driven by electrostatic-charged armor, spiritual states, projections, transference, countertransference, ecstasy, desires, needs, *Eros*, and love. By cultivating an unconditional regard toward anything that arises, all aspects of you become a part of the evolution of your consciousness and leads to a permanent union between body, consciousness, and love.

Rather than being something to heal, fix, or get rid of, each issue that arises during *Stillness Touch* is a portal for embodying love.

Such a holding field engenders the safety, trust, protection, and containment needed to surrender to love.

Before you touch, you and your recipient mutually enter a holding space so that you both can be with everything that transpires. You both agree that whatever happens in this space is not carried over into the everyday world. A *Stillness Touch* session is not about a personal relationship no matter what arises; rather, it is a spiritual practice for the evolution of consciousness. Therefore, whatever occurs in sacred space is not projected out; hold awareness inside so it develops as a potency within.

TRUST

The recipient is in total charge of the following aspects of the session: the intensity, intimacy, paradox gradient, and the physical touch boundaries. It all depends on a recipient's history, their capacity to trust the touch process and themselves, and to trust you, the practitioner, when you touch them. Both the one offering and the one receiving touch realize authentic boundaries by accessing the sensations that arise in the inner body, and by letting the qualities therein be the guide in determining how potent an intensity, intimacy, and paradox edge that each can be with. For example, the presence of electrically charged inner body static is an indicator for the practitioner to increase his *inner* body sensing presence. With a slower inner tempo, you can maintain a micro-discernment of the subtle nuances of inner body sensation that pulse as tones inside you that, by entrainment, transmit to the recipient who can do the same. Discomfort when intensity, intimacy, or paradox arises, does **not** mean anything needs to shift, although it does present us with the challenge to be with it.

A PRACTITIONER'S SELF-INQUIRY INTO ETHICS

When offering *Stillness Touch*, we are a fierce guardian of the recipient's tenuous unexpressed authentic boundaries. While touching your recipient, ask yourself:

"Do I separate myself from the recipient by objectification or efference?"

"Do I mind my boundaries?"

"Do I desire for something to happen for the recipient?"

"Do I push the recipient to go deeper?"

"Am I looking for the cranial wave, a tide, or primary respiration to appear?"

"Do I wish for the recipient to go into stillness, or do I inwardly suggest it?"

"Do I fear something may go wrong during the session?"

"What if something intense happens that I cannot handle?"

Catch the endless array of mental agendas and do not let thoughts or emotions 'behave' you, nor guide your touch during a session. Instead, repeatedly return to a neutral disposition, rest inward at the back of the heart, repose in *Eros* that wells from your pelvis, surrender to non-doing, and let yourself be guided by your inner body sensations in 'don't know.' From this neutral disposition, intensity, intimacy, and paradox self-resolves into stillness and will express as a whole-body pulse, *Spanda*, which indicates you may continue your touch. Be clear that you serve your client without harboring any personal agenda, a goal, or a need for any outcome, and do not operate out of fear or desires that come from unconscious drives.[54]

Stillness Touch empowers a recipient to navigate the embodiment of love.

It is prudent to offer a non-doing touch amid 'don't know' while reposing in a moment-by-moment inner sensing that connects you with your authentic boundaries that are guided by love. Maintain body-felt contact with your inner body stillness that naturally slows your inner body tempo of sensing. A whole-body felt-sense engenders a continuity of consciousness that streams as free attention that flows with love. Where and how to touch is based on your body felt-sense of the inner nuances of sensation, instead of being controlled by efference, agenda, treatment skills, ego, ideas, feelings, emotions, and your unconscious drives based on the past.

Now let's connect the dots between the practice of cranial work as a treatment therapy to the practice of *Stillness Touch* that is for the evolution of consciousness.

9

PRE-BIODYNAMIC, BIODYNAMIC, AND POST-BIODYNAMIC

L et us connect some dots between Pre-biodynamic, Biodynamic, and Post-biodynamic practices, with the understanding that words do not represent the realized body-felt experience. Words are a map, not the experience; have you ever used a map and gotten lost on a hiking trail? If yes, then you will appreciate the perspective that the map is an imperfect navigation system because it is not the actual territory we encounter in an embodied life, yet maps do provide a context. In the Dynamic Stillness School, we do not use words in place of the body-felt experience because, as Alfred Korzybski pointed out in his book *Science and Sanity*, "words are not the things."

Similarly, there is the danger of bypassing if biodynamic terms are a substitute for the actual realizations, which is a misuse of the Buddhist principle of right speech. When we characterize our living body-felt sense experiences in sensual body-felt language, it is a discipline that ensures we are not engaged in bypass, which again, occurs when we use terms in place of a living contact with a deeper reality. Why? Because slinging around jargon as though it is the actual felt-embodied realization creates a virtual reality in the mind. It confuses what Dr. Sutherland taught us that intellectual understanding is not the realized experience.

This misperception exists in the biodynamics outside of the osteopathic cranial field, and it is rampant within the spiritual traditions. For example, the repetition of mantrums is conflated with the experience of the level of consciousness that the mantra represents. That is why in every Dynamic Stillness school training, we ask participants to refrain from using terms, and instead to characterize the sensual qualities of their inner body-felt experience. Then we can place where our embodied living encounters with Breath of Life fit on the biodynamic map. When someone is interested in the map, we can connect the classical biodynamic terms with our actual body-felt experiences, and as a side benefit the map becomes more accurate.

The book *Stillness* connects inner body-felt experiences to terms in three ways: it provides cranial history as context; it presents the map, which are the precise osteopathic definitions that distinguish the three types of cranial work as crafted by Dr. Sutherland and the founding cranial osteopaths. Finally, *Stillness* characterizes in sensual language the qualities of living, embodied, felt-sense encounters with the tides. The realization of these domains of consciousness is required to transmit the potent expressions of life-force to others through touch. With that background in mind, let's explore how pre-biodynamic, biodynamic, and post-biodynamic terms fit together with our body-felt experience. Be forewarned; this will not be a linear presentation.

PRE-BIODYNAMIC: THE CRANIAL WAVE

In the Cranial Wave, consciousness is held inside the skin and is under the control of a narcissistic ego that is guided by the past and future.

The cranial wave rhythm has an unstable rate because its pulse changes according to the nervous systems' reaction to the stresses of life. The cranial wave is a record of our encounters with the stresses of life. Holographic patterns that are encoded by the limbic system are laid down in the tissues and distributed throughout the body as armor. Austrian M.D. Wilhelm Reich documented the distributions of body armor and assigned five behavior types of recoil to specific patterns: *schizoid, oral, masochist, psychopath,* and *rigid.* The cranial wave patterns that arise from trauma in the past create armor in the tissues, which are called lesion patterns in functional cranial work.

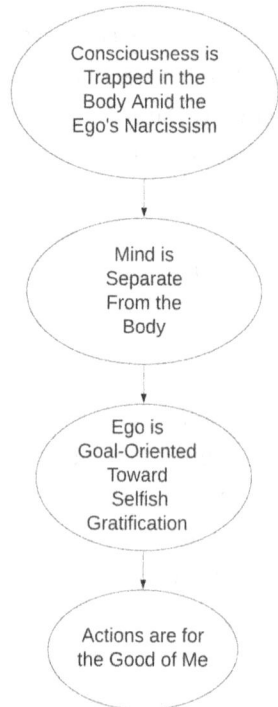

Consciousness is Trapped in the Body Amid the Ego's Narcissism

↓

Mind is Separate From the Body

↓

Ego is Goal-Oriented Toward Selfish Gratification

↓

Actions are for the Good of Me

Figure 8. Pre-Biodynamic

Cranial wave does not reveal the flow of life in the present; rather its patterns represent the impediments to life's flow that occurred in the past.

Cranial wave's holographic patterns record all the painful instances in which the flow of life, the *Tao*, did not go 'my way.'

The way of the narcissist demands that life serves me, which is the opposite of *Tao* that serves the whole. Ego manipulates life for its own gain, and when life unfolds differently from what the ego expected, we suffer. Ego maintains a narcissistic grip on our awareness that is strengthened by the emotionality of doubt, hatred, and fear. The subsequent trapped awareness deepens the ego's sense of separation that recoils our awareness from love. Some cranial practitioners can read your past from the cranial wave and can tell you when and how you had a specific injury.

> *The cranial wave is not a biodynamic tide. It is an ego-driven, nervous-system controlled enfoldment of everyday consciousness.*

A biodynamic session does not begin until the cranial wave disappears, which occurs after the practitioner and client realize neutral, marked by a sense of a whole-body stillness within which a whole-body breathing field arises. Neutral is the moment when stillness fills the whole body, and the potency of primary respiration transcends the ego and nervous system's control over the body. Here, in neutral, the heart field emanates the *presence of stillness* that conveys the realization that the body is a whole unit. Once this state of neutral arrives, we enter the biodynamic domain.

BIODYNAMIC: THE TIDES AND DYNAMIC STILLNESS

When contact with the *presence of stillness* places you in a neutral contact with the fluid tide and the long tide that dissolves in Dynamic Stillness, consciousness begins its *Ascending Journey* that leads to freedom from the ego's narcissism, as you can see below in Figure 9:

Here, in the biodynamic domain, we sense a breath-like welling and receding of consciousness inside our whole inner-body space, which is called primary respiration. It is considered primary because it is the breathing power of life that makes the body - an embryological force that is prior to the creation of anatomy, or a nervous system.

When stillness fills the body, and extends slightly beyond the skin and primary respiration starts to breathe, it is called the fluid tide. Then, with repeated contact, the fluid tide neutral deepens, and stillness will expand and pervade the body, the room, and the surrounding biosphere while primary respiration extends our consciousness to the edge of our known. This global *presence of stillness* is a neutral that expresses a vast, transpersonal, luminous breathing field called the long tide.

In contrast, the cranial wave is a condensing force that separates, while the potency of the ascending currents of the Breath of Life - as fluid tide and long tide - expands your awareness, frees it from ego's trap of narcissism, releases the nervous system control over the body, all of which leads you to the realization of the states of consciousness that are

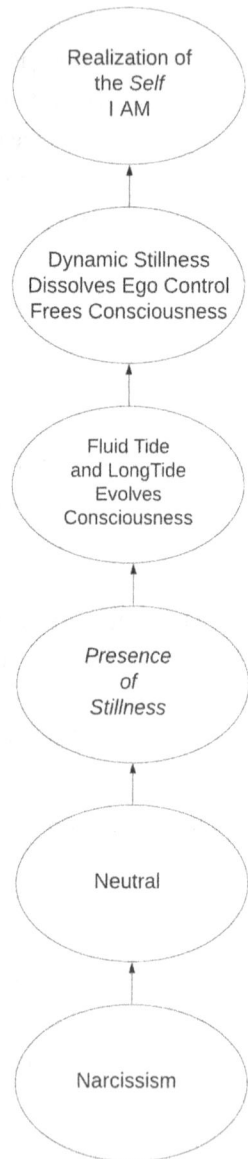

Realization of
the *Self*
I AM

↑

Dynamic Stillness
Dissolves Ego Control
Frees Consciousness

↑

Fluid Tide
and LongTide
Evolves
Consciousness

↑

Presence
of
Stillness

↑

Neutral

↑

Narcissism

Figure 9. Biodynamic

170

documented in the ancient spiritual traditions.

Both aspects of primary respiration - the fractal whole-body breathing field of the fluid tide and the vast global luminous breath of the long tide - impact the cerebrospinal fluid (CSF). The tides are aspects of the ascending life current that contain the forces of levity that lift and expand consciousness, freeing it from the gravitational pull of the ego's self-centering grip. Both the whole-body fluid and the global luminous tides express and resonate inside the CSF and are in harmony with the pulse of the heart's sinoatrial node. Stillness Touch practitioners repose directly in the source of this tidal CSF movement, which is within the pulsation at the heart's SA Node.

Touch offered amid an inner orientation of presence toward the SA Node facilitates in the recipient the realization of the tides as ever-expanding states of consciousness.

If the long tide neutral continues to deepen, our previous sense that the body is separate from everything in creation disappears. All that remains is black emptiness, the full-void that is called Dynamic Stillness. This is THE neutral, the source of neutral, which the Buddhists call the *Clear Light*.

Once we realize, or, better yet, once consciousness is engulfed by infinite black stillness, all sense of separation disappears between body, self, time, space, in, out, the *Self* and other - it all dissolves in an infinite black emptiness as a unified consciousness.

When infinite black stillness implodes in our inner-body space, we contact an inner infinity that is known in the Vedic tradition as the *Shiva*, which is Pure Consciousness, that inwardly suffuses awareness so thoroughly that it becomes our consciousness. In Jung's depth psychology and in the Vedic tradition, this is known as the realization of the *Self*, or I AM. If we can bear to realize our *Self*, which is our consciousness in its most refined form, then we enjoy a total bodily integration of all prior realized states of consciousness that range from the cranial wave to the long tide. Realization of the *Self* is the fruit of the ascending current.

Due to the mutuality that you and your recipient have established in neutral, you both can simultaneously realize ever-evolving states of consciousness during a *Stillness Touch* session. As a practitioner, you realize the evolutionary potential of all the frequencies of consciousness that resonate in the CSF through the power of neutral human touch. These realizations are transmitted both to you and the recipient through touch by the laws of entrainment. The realization of so-called exalted spiritual states is not a dream or abstraction, it is your natural state and birthright. Over time, the potency of Dynamic Stillness builds and implodes as an inner infinity within your body. This is a fulcrum for the descending current that suffuses consciousness in the cells.

POST-BIODYNAMIC: THE DESCENDING CURRENT OF LOVE IMPLODES INTO THE CELLS OF THE FLESH

After Dynamic Stillness descends to implode within the cells, all your previously realized states of consciousness combine as one and become a mysterious 'non-separating' super substance called the *Pure Breath of Love*. *Pure Breath of Love* suffuses the cells, all distinct tides disappear, and we enter a mapless post-biodynamic domain.

Again, once we enjoy the integration of *Pure Breath of Love*, we can no longer sense the tides as distinct enfoldments. Rather, we sense in all cells a whole-body pulse that is in tandem with the heartbeat. At *Pure Breath of Love,* the entire biodynamic map dissolves, which is why this is a post-biodynamic realization.

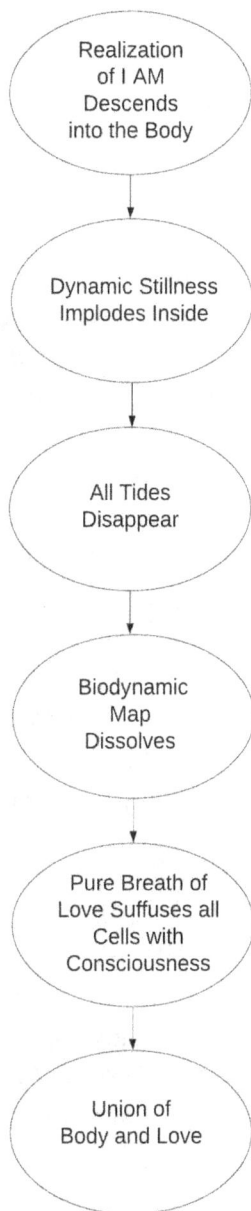

Figure 10. Post-Biodynamic

One student who realized Pure Breath of Love in a class said, "This isn't biodynamic cranial work anymore, is it?"

Above, Figure 10 outlines how the Descending Current leads consciousness from infinity into the cells of the body to the Enfleshment of *Pure Breath of Love*.

In *Pure Breath of Love*, we sense a singular substance that is an alchemical mix of all states of consciousness. The *Presence of Stillness* always accompanies *Pure Breath of Love* as a permanent seal of imploded Dynamic Stillness that *descends* to suffuse all the cells of the body with consciousness. The body now expresses an entirely new dimension of realization that co-breathes love within all of your cells, radiantly awakening each cell to full consciousness. At the Dynamic Stillness School, we realize that in *Pure Breath of Love* there is no line of separation between any harmonic of consciousness. Even though we have entered a post-biodynamic realm and the tides are no longer present, we can still recognize each stage of the biodynamic map to help the ego bear the uncomfortable reality of enflesh-ment, which occurs after *Pure Breath of Love* suffuses all of our cells.

An unbearable reality to the ego is there is no separation.

Everything is interconnected: the tides and all states of consciousness are seamlessly united as one. Once we realize the ever-evolving mystery of *Pure Breath of Love*, we experience that our *body is* the love that creates all that is.

Nothing is separate from love, no matter how uncomfortable, or how it appears.

Here, amid *Pure Breath of Love* during a *Stillness Touch* session, a practitioner is inwardly centered in the SA Node of the heart while reposed in *Eros* in the pelvis *as* primordial awareness with free attention. You are simply present *as* your state, while in neutral hand contact with the recipient. There is no search for the "perfect contact" or a treatment sequence. Instead, as a practitioner, you repose in Divine Ignorance while touching *as* neutral that naturally synchronizes with *Pure Breath of Love*.

As mentioned, the book *Stillness* characterizes the journey of the ascending life current to the heart radiance, which the *Taoists* call the *Shen*, that emanates as the pulse of the heart's SA node. When you offer neutral touch while abiding in *Shen*, it invokes the laws of entrainment that transmit the evolution of consciousness to a recipient. Chapter 9 of *Stillness* introduces an enfoldment previously undocumented in biodynamics that we now call *Pure Breath of Love*. This is a descending current of the evolution of consciousness that leads to the realization of the enfleshment of love.

Dynamic Stillness School graduates thoroughly explore this descending current as *Pure Breath of Love* descends into all the cells of the body and unites with the heart's self-existing radiance and with *Eros* in the pelvis.

Summary: The ignition of *Pure Breath of Love* creates a profound union between body, consciousness, the heart of mother earth, universal consciousness, and the tender mother love that creates all that is. This enfleshment of the Divine Feminine Will or *Pure Breath of Love*, contains the ascending tidal expressions of consciousness that utterly frees awareness from ego's narcissistic grip, and then combines the tidal life currents during the descent of consciousness into the body while love *enfleshes* all the cells.[55] In the spiritual traditions, the realization of the Divine Will is known as the *Completion Stage*, which implies an utter cellular suffusion of the superradiance of love that is a permanent union with The All. Enfleshment frees trapped *Eros* and relaxes the emotion-laden armor in the body, which when liberated transmutes into what the Buddhists call *innate bliss*. *Innate bliss* illuminates all recoils: everything remaining in you that impedes the evolution of your consciousness or thwarts your utter bodily union with love.

EVOLUTION OF CONSCIOUSNESS

To repeat, the above events do not occur in the order that I described them. It is only on a map that the neutral is preliminary to stillness, and whole-body stillness is prior to primary respiration. That is not what unfolds during *Stillness Touch* sessions with a living human being. The realization of living territory cannot be logically mapped and frozen into neat sequences, given the chaotic expression of simultaneous multiple states of consciousness that is our spectral body. We map the process only to help our ego feel comfortable amid the extremely uncomfortable, messy, unbearable chaos that is our fully lived reality as a spectral human being. However, at some point in our evolution, the map will have to go if we long for union with love.

> How much an ego needs comfort amid the chaos of intensity, intimacy, and paradox is the degree to which it needs a map to shield itself from feeling the harsh reality that occurs when life does not go 'my' way.

Since *Stillness Touch* is explicitly a path for the evolution of consciousness, we do not concern ourselves with naming tides or using cranial jargon. If we immerse our attention inward during our daily *Stillness Practices*, it is possible to repose in *Pure Breath of Love* and withstand its uncomfortable, messy, chaotic, intense, intimate, erotic, and paradoxical qualities. We repose in black stillness inside the body while sensing the qualities of the sensations therein. Recall from the book *Stillness* that inner sensing is our indigenous root function of the heart field as our organ of perception that is inherently united with nature.

Abrams characterized that by accessing our heart perception the *Flesh* of the world converses with our *flesh*, using nature's language without words.[56]

> When *Eros,* as the wisdom of the body, unites with *Sophia* as the World Wisdom, we enjoy one seamless breathing fractal flow of love that creates all things.

EROS IS YOUR WILL

Recall that even subtle acts of efference suppress the expression of the Divine Feminine within you, which adversely impacts your will, life force, *Eros, Prana, Shakti, chi,* whatever the name. When efference diminishes your will power, it hinders the evolution of your consciousness. *Eros,* life force, or will is the creative drive to wholeness. In neutral, we synchronize with life's potency, and our will naturally yields to the Will of the Divine Feminine.

> *You cannot unite with the Divine Feminine Will without first having freed your Eros so that it belongs to you.*

In place of letting Divine Feminine Wisdom, *Shakti,* or *Eros* guide us, ego employs thinking that assumes a false sovereignty over our body and will. As a result, we live life severed from a body-felt relationship with *Eros,* Nature, and Love. These are symptoms of the *Core Erotic Wound,* which occur early in life as the first event that separated us from our connection with *Eros,* the flow of love in the body. When we are suffering the *core wound* our thinking, feeling, and will are embroiled in an inner war. We feel separate from ourselves, others, and nature, and we may feel broken, deficient, alone, lost, confused, and disconnected from the wholeness of life, and bereft of love that creates all that is. When your *Eros* belongs to you, a soulful relatedness is possible *Eros*-to-*Eros* between two people that unites them with the love that creates all that is.

When *Eros* is free, our attention flows with and serves *Pure Breath of Love*. As mentioned, freed *Eros* enhances the potency of *innate bliss* that softens the body armor and releases the accumulated emotions, electricity, and shock in the flesh, which further strengthens your will. Eros, life force, *chi, prana, Shakti,* wisdom of the body, *innate bliss,* etc., again, these are different names for your will, your sacred power that is already one with the Divine Feminine Will.

> When your will is free from ego's grip, it unites with Divine Feminine Will.

LOVE IS THE SOURCE FOR THE POTENCY OF YOUR WILL

By daily engaging the descending current during your *Stillness Practice,* your *Eros* gradually becomes free. After the softening of your body armor and the release of past emotions, electricity, shock, and trauma from your flesh, you acclimate to the increased potency of *Eros* that surges powerfully throughout your body. Given that your will is an expression of the love that creates all that is, you not only realize what your life's purpose is, you effortlessly achieve it.

> Your talk becomes a walk that is suffused with love for the rest of your life. You effortlessly express the unique gifts that you

are here to manifest. When your 'talk is walk' it means your three centers have united.

THREE PRIMARY BODY CENTERS: HEAD, HEART, PELVIS

When the three primary body centers, head, heart, and pelvis, evolve and mature they become 'three hearts' that then unify to become one heart, which pulses as love in each cell. Some spiritual traditions insist that the seven hearts become one, correlating each heart with the seven major chakra centers in the body. Although true, in Figure 11 we navigate the qualities in the three primary centers:

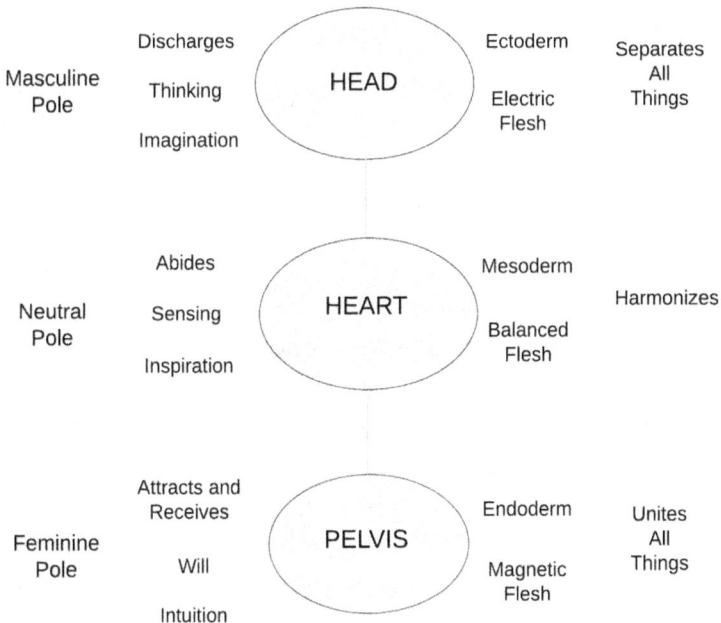

Masculine Pole	Discharges Thinking Imagination	HEAD	Ectoderm Electric Flesh	Separates All Things
Neutral Pole	Abides Sensing Inspiration	HEART	Mesoderm Balanced Flesh	Harmonizes
Feminine Pole	Attracts and Receives Will Intuition	PELVIS	Endoderm Magnetic Flesh	Unites All Things

Figure 11. Three Primary Centers

STILLNESS PRACTICE UNITES THE THREE CENTERS AS ONE

Practice: Abide inwardly *as* the self-existing radiance of your heart while reposed in the *Eros* of your pelvis that connects with the heart of the mother earth, which is already united with Pure Consciousness and Universal Love. *Eros*, trapped as armor in your flesh, is freed, which softens the armor and releases the trapped electricity, shock, and emotionality in your flesh, which, again, strengthens your will.

Your strength of will becomes so unwavering that it permanently reconnects *Eros* in the pelvis with the self-existing heart radiance, and together they unite with the pulsing heart of mother earth that expresses Pure Consciousness and the Love of the Whole.

After you establish the pelvis as the seat of personal will, and you can repose here, your will spontaneously unites with the Will of the Divine Feminine, and you realize *Not my will, but Thine.*

When you are united with Divine Feminine Will, the subsequent descending life current implodes and suffuses love so deep into all your cells that the bottom drops out, and you discover an inner-body infinity. It is similar to when the ascending life current implodes at the heart's SA Node that leads to the realization of the heart's infinite self-existing radiance that is known as *Shen*. Except here, when the bottom drops out in your pelvis, you forever unite your *Eros* with *Pure Breath of Love*. Amid this permanent utter bodily union with love, there is no perceivable difference between love and your body. We call this enfleshment.

REALIZED INNER QUALITIES OF ENFLESHMENT

In enfleshment, love suffuses every cell, radiantly awakening them into the *Completion Stage*. Enfleshment is the result of being so still that the descending current of love implodes within, which permanently ends your inner war. Recall that the inner war manifests due to conflicts between the three primary body centers in the head, heart, and pelvis. Each battle blocks the inner body flow of *Eros* and creates knots that recoil awareness from love. In Enfleshment, the inner war resolves, *Eros* pulses freely, and reunites the three centers that pulse *Pure Breath of Love* as One Heart:

Will: *Sacred Pulse of Love* is the Divine Feminine Will that moves your body.

Feeling: *The Sacred Sense of Love* erotically connects you to everything.

Thinking: *Cosmic Love* imagines your thoughts.

Notice above, that there is a subtle life-changing event called the 'reversed will.'

Here, the will is in charge as guided by the Divine Feminine Will, and thinking follows along. Whereas prior to the cellular implosion of love, thinking dictated the will, and we acted as directed by the thinking ego.

Although enfleshment is mapless, when you consciously traverse the classical biodynamic ascending tidal map it provides insight into the fundamental mysteries of a mapless enfleshment. Dynamic Stillness, now always present, seals and protects from harm all enfoldments and frequencies of consciousness. Each enfoldment of consciousness is integral to the mapless domain of enfleshment. Below are the qualities that indicate a realization of the *Completion Stage*.

BOTH/AND

You realize a full spectrum paradoxical existence *both* as a human limited by your givenness, *and* as a boundless spiritual being. All aspects of self and *Self* are included, nothing is left out, and you can effortlessly be with all of you, as you are, without trying to change the shadow aspects in yourself, in others, or life. You realize and embody Divine Repose, which means you can let everything in life unfold as it is.

'THE ALL' EXPRESSES THE PRESENCE OF STILLNESS

All tidal expressions of consciousness harmonically coexist as one alchemical substance that is sealed inside Dynamic Stillness. The *Presence of Stillness* contains all qualities and yet no single quality is discernible. Again, Jung calls this realm the *Pleroma*.

IN THIS POST-BIODYNAMIC REALM, THE BIODYNAMIC MAP DISAPPEARS

The classical biodynamic map dissolves, meaning the tides are no longer perceivable as discrete expressions of consciousness during meditation or while offering *Stillness Touch*. All that remains is black stillness within which pulses *Pure Breath of Love* in every cell of the body in tandem with the heartbeat. This paradoxical domain of The *Great Black Mother* is not mappable.

A SENSUOUS BODILY CONNECTION WITH EVERYTHING

You feel erotically connected to nature, events, places, people, states, and dimensions. No words convey the degree of absolute relatedness that expresses as an erotic bodily union with 'the All.' Enfleshment becomes your ordinary state of consciousness.

A SENSE OF A NON-SEPARATING MATTER THAT UNIFIES

Rather than feeling separated into discrete parts, all aspects of you function harmoniously as one. You sense union down into every cell while feeling continuously suffused by a mysterious, invisible 'non-separating' matter. The pulse of this non-separating liquid crystal super substance emanates the essence of the heart as *Shen*. This is a superradiance of love that makes you whole and erotically connects you with everything. There is no ability to sense separation from love, except as an observation by the ego of the surface appearance of things.

Your ego's capacity to separate is gone. If 'separation' occurs, it is based on a remembrance of the past when your life was under the control of ego's separating self-sense.

FREE

Being inexorably bodily united with the love that creates all that is, your will is utterly free. No event, person, psychological complex, and no outside force can compel you to action. Your will is so free that you are moved to act only by love.

BODY AS LOVE

Every cell is suffused by, and in sensuous union with the love that creates all that is - this is not revocable.

If love moves, so your body moves as its expression.

YOU ARE FREE FROM YOUR EGO'S FALSE SENSE OF SEPARATION

Your hidden compulsive thoughts, drives, impulses, and psychological complexes that previously moved you to action no longer have the power to control your will and ruin your life. You effortlessly flow in the river of your *Tao* while reposed on a magic carpet.

FREEDOM IS ORDINARY

Once you acclimate to enfleshment, you enjoy utter freedom from outside influences as your everyday consciousness. Your freedom is unwavering, as a realization of a permanent all-cell bodily union with love that creates all that is.

THE GREAT DISSOLUTION BEYOND DYNAMIC STILLNESS

Then, as mentioned, another implosion, better characterized as an utter exhaustion occurs. When this utter exhaustion completes itself, it dissolves everything that is unaligned with the fundamental reality of your natural state of union. Softly and imperceptibly every recoil from love disappears into thin air, including all that you cherish, the near and dear, avoided, feared, and dreaded. What also dissolves are the power of old attachments, reifications, the self-hated aspects of your personality. Even gone is your pride of intellect, the enamor of your profound and exalted spiritual realizations, the numinous states, the gratification of your worldly accomplishments, ambitions, your desires for the accumulation of wealth, social status, possessions, homes. The precious and the dreaded and revolted, all of what you previously felt were essential or you hated, its power over you dissolves into nothing.

YOU DO NOT MOVE UNLESS LOVE MOVES YOU

To reemphasize, this dissolution takes with it everything, including the remnants of your exalted spiritual states. Even the importance of your consciousness dissolves. What is left is ordinary simplicity. In Buddhism, it is called *suchness*, it is *just so*, or *tathata*. Zen calls this the realization of the Tenth Bull or *Zhenrin*: you are a genuine person who reenters the marketplace completely ordinary.

> "Then I came back from where I'd been. My room, it looked the same. But there was nothing left between the Nameless and the named."[57]

AN UTTER REPOSE IN DIVINE IGNORANCE

> Everything is what it is - as it is - with no capacity to embellish life in any way.

You can no longer project extra meaning, cosmic implications, fantasy, magical thinking, glamour, or any other special bigger-than-life qualities, nor make exalted claims of synchronistic events, enlightened people, places, or experiences.

Everything dissolves and collapses into the ordinary in the most literal sense. This is not profound ordinariness; it is just ordinary.

BE STILL AND KNOW I AM LOVE

APPENDIX 1

SPIRITUAL TRADITIONS AND THE HEART'S
SELF-EXISTING RADIANCE

The heart is the center of the human being where spirit and flesh interface.

THE WISDOM OF THE HEART

The spiritual paths sighted below emphasize the practice of *Pratyahara*, which means to orient your awareness inward to sense the divine radiant qualities of your heart field. *Pratyahara* unites body, consciousness, and love, which you realize when you abandon the fear-based controlling strategies of recoil from the ego that drives your attention and will outward. You may recall that efference over-wills the natural inner-body flow of the *Tao*. That is because the ego wants its way; it wants to be in charge and control life by using efference to externalize attention, objectify, and separate due to its need to fix, modify, name, and to know. Ego avoids uncomfortable qualities that arise during *Stillness Practices* or *Touch*; therefore, a crucial practice, instead of letting ego control your will, see if you can surrender to the Divine Will. Orient to an inner-body sensing and let the sensations therein guide your awareness that arise from the body's wisdom.

The wisdom of your body is one with the Wisdom of the Whole.

We have reviewed the non-doing principles that Dr. Sutherland gave to us, which Dr. Becker coined as biodynamics, and now we can appreciate that the heart is an organ of perception that evolves consciousness.

The quotes below were compiled by Kurt Keutzer, PhD for the *Stillness Touch* Lay Courses with my gratitude. These excerpts are from spiritual traditions that recognize the heart's SA Node as the center of primordial consciousness, the *Self*, or I AM.

VEDIC UPANISHADS: PURUSHA, ANGUSHTAMATRA.

Katha Upanishad Tr. by Vidyavachaspati V. Panoli

The *Purusha* of the size of a thumb dwells in the heart. Realizing the Lord of the past and the future, one does not need to protect oneself. This verily is that which thou seekest. *Purusha* is defined as the Universal Principle that is eternal, indestructible, without form, and all-pervasive (2-I-12).

The *Purusha* of the size of a thumb is like a smokeless flame and is the Lord of the past and the future. Purusha certainly exists now and shall certainly exist tomorrow. This verily is that which thou seekest (2-I-12).

Purusha of the size of a thumb is the inner Self that is ever seated in the heart of all living beings. One should, with steadiness, know Him as pure and immortal (2-III-17). *Katha Upanishad* Tr. By Vidyavachaspati V. Panoli

Svetasvatara Upanishad - Tr. by Swami Tyagisananda.

The *Angushtamatra* assumes a form the size of a thumb, by virtue of intellect, emotion, imagination, and will. The Infinite Being dwells in the heart as the inner Self. Those who realize this become immortal (III-12).

Infinite Being has a thousand heads, a thousand eyes, and a thousand feet enveloping the whole universe (III-14).

Subtle as the point of a goad, and pure, effulgent, and infinite like the sun, *Angushtamatra* alone is seen assuming as another the size of a thumb on account of the finiteness of the heart in which He appears, and He associates Himself with egoism and *Sankalpa* on account of the limitations of the intellect (V-8). *Svetasvatara Upanishad* Tr. By Swami Tyagisananda.

HINDU: AYODHYA, SPANDA, SACRED TREMOR, DYNAMIC STILLNESS, SELF-EXISTING HEART RADIANCE, HRIDAYA, PRATYAHARA

From the viewpoint of yoga practice, the golden sheath of the divine city, *Ayodhya*, which is a mass of light-filled with bliss, has its abode in the subtle area of the grape-shaped hollow of the physical heart. It is in the castle of this causal sheath that the immortal individual soul abides with its supreme protector, all-powerful, omniscient, adorable father, God. The temple of a yogi is inside the heart alone.[58]

KASHMIR SHAIVISM: SPANDA, SACRED TREMOR, DYNAMIC STILLNESS

Kashmir Shaivism is near and dear to my heart because many biodynamic cranial principles are derived from it, as we will see. The heart's self-existing radiance that emanates from the pacemaker is known in Kashmir Shaivism as the *Spanda, Sacred*

Pulse, or the *Sacred Tremor*. One realizes *Spanda* by the inner body union of *Shiva* and *Shakti* during the practice of *pratyahara*, which as you recall, is the practice of orienting awareness inward to contact the divinity within (See Advaita below).

The pacemaker (SA Node) of the heartbeat is in the right atrium or the upper right chamber of the heart. It is here that the Radiant Transcendental Consciousness is continually associated with the impulse of Life in the individual body-mind. [59]

Swami Chetanananda Writes About Dr. Rollin Becker

> The fundamental energy of life has a spiral manifestation, what the osteopath Dr. Rollin Becker refers to as a spiral tide. It is actually a tide within a tide within a tide that continuously folds in on itself, which is why it is described as a serpent. This is not merely a metaphor, but a description of the actual experience. Our (inner-body) breathing of 12 times a minute constitutes a tide, within which there is a tide of the fluctuation of cerebrospinal fluid. Within that, there is yet another (deeper) tide. This spiral energy of *kundalini* is constantly unfolding and rising, then contracting and descending, and within that, there are other currents still. Relative to each (tidal) level of breath, there are corresponding levels (of consciousness), ... on one level we are attuning ourselves ... to *prana-kundalini*; here our sense of corporeal materiality dissolves and our awareness of (a breathing) flow takes over. We don't notice our bodies so much anymore. We can bring it to a stillpoint, it condenses and then goes quiet, and by following the energy to its source, we have access to the energy that powers our individualized consciousness, or *Chita-kundalini*, which we experience as the pulsation of the mind and emotions.[60]

DR. ROLLIN BECKER AND HIS CONNECTION TO KASHMIR SHAIVISM

The above is Swami Chetanananda's characterization of Dr. Becker's understanding of the principles of Kashmir Shaivism as it relates to biodynamics. Yet what follows is a mystery. Traditionally, US osteopaths do not air their spiritual beliefs publicly due to the harsh criticism from official 'medical' osteopathy, so I am grateful to Swami Khecaranatha (Nathaji) who lived at the Movement Center Ashram and shared his experiences with Dr. Becker. Nathaji is the author of several books on Kashmir Shaivism and is the founder of the spiritual center Rudramandir in Berkeley, California. Nathaji told me that a devotee who lived in the ashram, received regular sessions from Dr. Rollin Becker when he'd visit the ashram, the Movement Center in Portland, Oregon. He loved working with stillness so much that he introduced Dr. Becker to his guru Swami Chetanananda. There was an immediate mutual understanding and a meeting in the depths between Dr. Becker and Swami Chetanananda. Even though each had their own realizations, they found resonance, respect, and mutual recognition in Dynamic Stillness, which is also known in Kashmir Shaivism as the *Spanda*. It appears that the Swami coined Dynamic Stillness, and later Dr. Becker began to use it as a biodynamic cranial term.

Swami Chetanananda received sessions from Dr. Becker, and one time he said he experienced the embodied presence of Swami Nityananda, the guru of Chetanananda's guru Swami Rudrananda. On his Movement Center website, the Swami said, "Dr. Becker had a profound understanding of the potential that animates the human being and the process by which that potential transforms into physiology, cognition, and perception." Swami Chetanananda says that Dr. Becker taught him cranial osteopathy for many years and Swami dedicated his two books *Dynamic Stillness* Volumes 1 & 2 to Dr. Rollin Becker.

Dr. Becker gave sessions at the ashram until his passing in 1976. On the cover of Dr. Rollin Becker's Rudra Press book, *Life in Motion,* is a painting called *The Mobius Strip,* which is a sculpture in the garden at Swami Chetanananda's ashram. The Swami said that Dr. Rollin Becker's and his wife's ashes rest there. Dr. Rachael Brooks, who lived at Swami Chetanananda's ashram, trained with Becker and edited his books, *Life in Motion* and *Stillness in Life.* Brooks also edited Dr. Sutherland's book, *Teaching in the Science of Osteopathy.* All three books were published by Rudra Press, the ashram's imprint.

ADVAITA: HRIDAYA, PRATYAHARA

Paraphrasing the qualities of the ascending life current by master Ramana Maharshi, "the godly atom of the Self is to be found in the right chamber of the heart, (SA Node). Here lies the Heart, the dynamic Spiritual Heart called *hridaya,* located on the right side of the heart that is clearly visible to the inner eye of an adept on the Spiritual Path. Through meditation, you can learn to find the Self in the cave of the Heart."

Pratyahara: when you orient your sensing awareness inward toward your midline, known in Advaita as *pratyahara,* it means to withdraw the primary focus of attention from the external senses to the internal. While practicing *pratyahara,* a realization occurs after your inner sensuality expands your perception inward: it becomes a divine perception filled with inner ecstasy. When your inner divine sensuality expands back out into the everyday world, you enjoy erotic divine perception everywhere.

CHRISTIAN: THE HOLY BREATH OF SOPHIA, EYE OF THE HEART, NOUS

"Love is the very physical structure of the universe, driving all things toward union, attraction, and cosmic sympathy," says Teilhard de Chardin. Dr. de Chardin also notes that there is a sensual longing for communion with others who have this larger vision of Love. The immense fulfillment of the friendships between those engaged in furthering the evolution of consciousness has a quality almost impossible to describe.

Esoteric Christian traditions teach that when you orient attention toward the innerness, you contact the *Holy Breath of Sophia* that unites all things. When *Sophia* is present, the "two become one, inner becomes outer, and outer becomes inner."

The Christian Fathers of the Desert characterized the heart as not simply a physical organ; it is also the spiritual center of the human being. The heart is our deepest and truest Self, the inner shrine to be entered only through the sacrifice of ego, and in which the mystery of the union between the divine and the human occurs. The Desert Fathers say the heart is an organ of contemplation, the *Eye of the Heart*, or *Nous*. The *Nous* dwells in the depths of the soul and represents the innermost aspect of the heart. *Nous*, the *Eye of the Heart*, is the highest faculty of man by which one knows God. With *Nous* you can realize the inner essences of each of the 12 Spiritual Hierarchies, using the spiritual perception as a direct apprehension of the heart.

"God is born in the Heart, and the Heart is born in God."
~ Meister Eckhart

ISLAM: EYE OF THE HEART

Sufi

Sufi's sacred symbol is a winged heart within which are a five-pointed star and the crescent moon under the star. The star represents divine light, and the moon is the responsiveness to the light. Sufi Master Hazrat Inayat Khan says, "In the deepest depth of the heart is the voice of the spirit."

The *Eye of the Heart* is also a motif in the Sufi tradition. To a Sufi, the heart is the door to the Divine, the eye through which you see the depth of the heart, and through which the heart can know the Supreme Divine Reality. The *Eye of the Heart* operates in two dimensions at the same time: one eye orients toward the "interior" through which the meditator can sense the infinite depths of divinity within the heart, and the other eye orients toward the "exterior." This multidimensional eye is our lens through which the Supreme Subject, the Inner Knower, God, or primordial consciousness beholds the world.

> "I am contained neither in my sky nor my earth, but I am contained in the heart of the devoted." ~ Shams-i-Tabrizi

BUDDHISM: PRAJNAPARAMITA, TSONG GANG, UNBORN BUDDHA-MIND, MAHAMUDRA, INNATE BLISS, GREAT BLISS, AND THE GREAT SEAL OF PERFECTION.

Dzogchen

Tsong gang is formless primordial wisdom that is beyond form, shape, and color. It is inexpressible primordial wisdom beyond letters, words, and names. Non-conceptual primordial wisdom is beyond the concepts and discernment of the mind. *Twenty-*

one Nails: Oral Tradition of Zhang-Zhung, Chapter 5: The Thumb-Sized Body of Wisdom.

Buddhists also call this principle *Prajnaparamita*, Wisdom of the Whole, Mother of all Buddhas, and *Unborn Buddha Mind*. It is the immortal principle that unites emptiness and form, or consciousness and love. Tantric Buddhism calls it *Mahamudra, Innate Bliss,* or *Great Bliss.*

Zen

Here is a paraphrased version of a fifteenth-century account of words spoken by the Zen master Bankei: "The unborn is the origin and beginning of all there is; no source is apart from it and there is no beginning that is before the unborn. Thought has fallen one or more removes from the living reality of the unborn. Because of the unborn-ness and marvelous illuminative power inherent in the unborn Buddha-mind, it readily reflects all things, and when a thought comes along, it transforms itself into them. This turns the unborn Buddha-mind into thought. It is only our ignorance of the unborn Buddha-mind that makes us go and transform it into thoughts … in the external world, … we turn the unborn into all manner of things, and then we become those things. You must thoroughly understand about not transforming the unborn Buddha-mind into other things. Therefore, whatever happens, leave things as they are; do not worry yourself over them, and do not side with yourself. Just stay as you are, right in the unborn Buddha-mind, and do not change it into something else. Resist the partiality for yourself, which makes you want to have things move in your own way."

TAOISM: SHEN, ZHENREN

Shen is a Taoist term that translates as Spirit; it is our conscious presence that lives in the heart as an aspect of our being by which we radiate our essence into the world. [61]

"The heart is the master of the body, and the shen is the treasure of the heart." ~ Jingshen, Huainanzi

"One commits oneself to *Tao* by decreasing, as a day by day removal of the obstructions that block the *Tao* until there is no doing, which leads to the perfected state *Zhenren*"

Now let's navigate the heart's pacemaker as the center of the human being.

APPENDIX 2

NAVIGATING THE SA NODE, THE
PACEMAKER OF THE HEART

The SA Node is navigated by inwardly orienting your attention backwards toward the spine with your body-felt-sense presence. Once you can effortlessly sense within the domain of the heart field, then uniting with your heart's self-existing radiance becomes instant - as an intuitive act of will that occurs as direct apprehension. After you bodily acclimate to the intense power of your heart's radiant qualities, your radiant *presence of stillness* becomes stable in your body and a new awareness dawns amid an expanded level of consciousness. Here, you realize that your body is whole as an infinite radiance.

Meanwhile, you can directly intuit the SA Node, but not as a physical place, nor as a contrived visualization of a point of radiant light, rather the body becomes an inner sense organ of infinite radiance that you effortlessly intuit in an instant. The realization of the whole-body as a sense organ replaces your previous self-identification that the physical body is limited. This realization arises due to directly accessing the point where the life current combines with the body before it distributes to the body: this place is the pacemaker, or SA Node.

The SA Node has an intrinsic rhythm that is directed by *Pure Breath of Love*. It is independent of the nervous system, brainwaves, tides, and body functions.

The SA Node is the primary fulcrum in the human being, and the connection point, the center, and source point, where the body receives the life currents; this is the seat of the *Self* in the body. Intrinsic impulses from the SA node cause the heartbeat, and *Pure of the Breath of Love* distributes the self-existing radiance of life into the entire body-mind.

The heart field's self-existing radiance emanates an unwavering *presence of stillness*, which is the portal that grants you access to the full range between the terrestrial and celestial domains. As you read in Appendix 1, Swami Yogeshwaranand Saraswati, Bubba Free John, the Desert Fathers, the Vedas, Sufi's, Taoists, Hindus, Buddhists, and others have written that the physical access point for the self-existing radiance of the heart is at the SA node, or pacemaker. In modern times, Sri Aurobindo, Rudolf Steiner, Saniel Bonder, and Neil Cohen have championed the heart as our center.

PRATYAHARA AS STILLNESS PRACTICE

Recall that a post-biodynamic *Stillness Touch* session is offered, while orienting your awareness within the heart field, which is the practice of *Pratyahara* (Advaita). You bask in the *presence of stillness* as your self-existing heart radiance at the SA node; also called the *Shen* (Taoism), *Purusha*, or *Angushtamatra* (Upanishads), which is the primordial wisdom, or *tshon gang* (Dzogchen). Once you land in your heart field, you also repose in your pelvic floor to sense *Eros*, or *innate bliss* (Buddhist Tantra).

The presence of *innate bliss* indicates that you have united your *Eros* with *Purusha, Shen,* or the self-existing radiance of your heart. Both the heart and pelvic essences are connected-as-one to the Etheric Heart of Mother Earth that unites pure consciousness with universal love. *Pure Breath of Love* is also known as the *Sacred Tremor,* or *Spanda* in Kashmir Shaivism, and it is *Prajnaparamita* in Buddhism.

You realize *Pure Breath of Love* after the vastness of the hearts' ever-expanding field touches infinity, extends beyond, and then implodes inside your body. Here, in the *inner* infinite stillness, *Pure Breath of Love* falls into itself, which is known as *rang 'babs* in Tibetan Buddhism, by pouring into and through *Purusha,* the thumb-sized primordial wisdom at the heart's sinoatrial node. *Pure Breath of Love* fills your infinite inner body space - that is the Pure Consciousness of Dynamic Stillness - as well as suffuses all of the body's cells with the dynamism of love. The cellular suffusion of *Pure Breath of Love* grants you an embodied realization of the *Great Bliss,* or *Mahamudra* as it is known in Buddhist Tantra. This is a primordial unity between the *yin* and *yang* that is called *Zhenren,* the perfected state, in Taoism.

When *Pure Breath of Love* expresses a whole-body pulse that is in unison with your heartbeat as *Spanda,* it indicates that you have entered what the Buddhists call the *Completion Stage* of realization. This is a non-mappable journey of permanent non-separation between body, consciousness, and love that creates all that is.

THE PRACTITIONER DISPOSITION IN PURE BREATH OF LOVE

In review, during a post-biodynamic *Stillness Touch* session, you offer touch *as* the self-existing radiance of heart's sinoatrial node, the *Angushtamatra* (Upanishads), which is the primordial wisdom, *tshon gang* (Dzogchen). Again, after heart radiance unites with the sensuousness of *Eros* that wells from the pelvis, it gives rise to *innate bliss*, which inherently connects to the heart of mother earth and unites pure consciousness with universal love, which is the Buddhist *Prajnaparamita*.

While reposing *as* this disposition, anywhere you place your hands on a recipient's body, there is the *Sacred Pulse* of the *Spanda* that tremors in tandem with your heartbeat.

REVIEW OF YOUR REALIZATIONS WITHIN PURE BREATH OF LOVE

You and the recipient are aware of the vastness of the *presence of stillness* as a conscious ever-expanding heart field that emanates radiance from the thumb-sized primordial wisdom at the SA node that is in union with *Eros* in the pelvis as *innate bliss*. Paradoxically however, the heart field is also always connected with the complete stillness, the exhaustion, or the emptiness at the heart's pacemaker - even though *Pure Breath of Love* has suffused the inner body and all your cells. The *Clear Light*, or Dynamic Stillness, is the infinite full void that seals and protects everything. Variously known as the *Great Seal of Perfection*, the *Great Bliss, Shen*, or *Mahamudra*, all enfoldments of consciousness are sealed inside Dynamic Stillness that form a precise alchemical mix of essential qualities of the five elements that combine to specifically evolve each recipient's consciousness. *Pure Breath of Love* is super radiant love that suffuses all cells and sensuously pulses with the heartbeat in union with The All.

GREAT SEAL AND GREAT PERFECTION

All emanations of consciousness are an aspect of *Pure Breath of Love* that is sealed in the *Clear Light*, or Dynamic Stillness, which again in Tibetan Buddhism is called the *Great Seal, Great Bliss*, or

Mahamudra. All emanations of consciousness are spontaneously perfected, matured, fructified and united as one to become the 'great perfection' or *Dzogchen*, which in Taoism is *Zhenrin.* Another way to characterize this realization is you are reposed in *Divine Ignorance* in a *Cloud of Unknowing.*

DIVINE IGNORANCE

"Divine ignorance means that you are ignorant in a Divine Way of everything in this universe. In other words, you become very humble and very truthful, when you realize you don't know what anything is. You have no idea in your mortal mind what anything is all about."[62] ~ Robert Adams

As with most spiritual practices, once you realize primordial awareness, which is the fruition of the ascending enfoldments of consciousness, you realize the *Self.* If you then decide to continue and descend into the body as the *Self,* the perspective dramatically changes.

With an inner body union between the self-existing radiance of heart and *Eros* in your pelvis, both the source and the fruition of the path unite, culminating as the realization of the *Great Bliss* (Tantric Buddhism).

From here, every skill previously learned and known by the practitioner dissolves and is left behind; you offer sessions in a Cloud of Unknowing, or Divine Ignorance. The classical biodynamic tidal map disappears, and the tides are no longer accessed individually, which is why it is considered post-biodynamic (See Chapter 7, *Realized Inner Qualities of Enfleshment*).

IN A POST-BIODYNAMIC JOURNEY INTO LOVE, THE BIODYNAMIC MAP DISSOLVES

As you recall, the classical biodynamic cranial map consists of the ascending currents fluid tide and long tide that culminate in the realization of Dynamic Stillness as the self-existing radiance of the heart at the SA node.

However, beyond Dynamic Stillness, the classical tidal map dissolves, and the steps of that path are left behind because the ascending map of the tides recedes into the background. The ascending path that the book *Stillness* presents in Chapters 5 through 8 leads to the realization of the *Self*, or I AM. This is a union of the body with pure consciousness that arises because of your regular daily *Stillness Practices* and by offering neutral *Stillness Touch.* The Sutherlands realized it as, Be Still And Know I AM.

Going further requires mutual participation between practitioner and recipient. Entry into the descending stream of *Pure Breath of Love* occurs by the interface between *Purusha*, which is the self-existing radiance of the heart, and the *innate bliss* of *Eros* in the pelvis. *Stillness Touch* is now a mapless post-biodynamic session that you offer with free attention. The practitioner abides as *Purusha, Shen,* the self-existing radiance of heart, while reposed as the *innate bliss* of *Eros* in the pelvis, which together emanate the superradiance of *Pure Breath of Love* that pulses within all cells in tandem with the heartbeat. The hands are in neutral contact with a recipient who is quietly receptive.

> Transmission occurs through neutral touch by the laws of entrainment. There is no need to do anything as a practitioner, other than *be.*

This is an endless descending life current journey into *Pure Breath of Love* with no map. Both the source and fruition of the path are realized as the inner-body union of self-existing heart radiance with *Eros* in the pelvis, which unites Pure Consciousness and Universal Love. Then the practice of *Stillness Touch* is remarkably simple:

> Fall into your awareness as a self-existing radiance that is united with Eros. Remain present as that awareness in neutral hand contact. Let the laws of entrainment take care of the rest.

For the well-seasoned, experienced, post-biodynamic practitioner, the entire path of attending to the classical enfoldments of the tidal map of fluid tide and long tide is dropped, and you simply:

"Fall into your own nature."
Tibetan "rang babs:" simply drop, babs, into yourself, rang.
"Be Still And Know I AM."

APPENDIX 3

QUOTES FROM OSTEOPATHS AND PHILOSOPHERS

The below quotes, with the references included, reflect the ancient spiritual traditions that we reviewed in Appendix 1.[63]

A.T. STILL, THE FOUNDER OF OSTEOPATHY.

The heart is the center of force and constructive intelligence in the body (*The Heart*, an article by A.T. Still, 1904).

First is formed the material heart, in which the spiritual establishes an office in which to dwell (*Philosophy and Mechanical Principles of Osteopathy*, 48).

The heart, not the brain, is the center and source of an intelligence that constructs each division of the body, and combines all parts into one common personage or being. There, we find the first movement of life in the embryo (A.T. Still, *Early Osteopathy in the Words of A. T. Still* 1991, 347).

She [the heart] is a graduate from the school of the Infinite, and her works are expected to show perfection in forethought, and are to be inspected, passed upon, received, or rejected by the scrutinizing mind of the Infinite (A.T. Still, *Autobiography of A. T. Still* 1908, 47).

The body is the second placenta. ~ A.T. Still

I find in man a miniature universe. I find matter, motion, and mind. When the elder prays, he speaks to God; he can conceive of nothing higher than mind, motion, and matter, the attributes of mind comprising love and all that pertains to it. In man, we find a complete universe (*Autobiography of A.T. Still,* 1908, 406).

In the union of any two elements we have a cause producing an effect, a new being superior to either element in the compound. Unite hydrogen with oxygen, the result is water, a new being. We find in man and beast that previous to the formation of a new being there must be a union of two lives...In the union of male and female elements we have a child (A.T. Still, *Osteopathy, Research and Practice.* 1910, 279).

The result is faultless perfection, because the earth-life shows in material forms the wisdom of the God of the celestial. Thus, we say biogen or dual life, that life means eternal reciprocity that permeates all nature. The celestial worlds of space or ether-life give forms wisely constructed...human life, in form and motion, is the result of conception by the terrestrial mother from the celestial father (A.T. Still, *The Philosophy and Mechanical Principles of Osteopathy* 1902, 251- 252).

THE THREE WISE MEN WHO TRANSMITTED OSTEOPATHY TO DR. STILL

Dr. Still had the sensation of being struck by a fist between the shoulders. Straightening up, he was made aware of the presence of three men from the unseen. They gave their names as Trali- ape, Trenagore, and Lahemphanen. They stated that they were

Egyptian philosophers and healers; that they had come to give him a new system of therapeutics. If he would fight the medical doctors, they would 'clear the driftwood' out of his way. ~ June 22, 1874, Addison Brewer

WILLIAM SUTHERLAND

Dr. Still could not speak of all the things he understood about the living human body. We were not ready to hear him (*Contributions of Thought - The Collected Writings of William Garner Sutherland, D.O.*, 1971, 293).

I have often said that we have lost something in osteopathy that Dr. Still tried to get across. That was the spiritual, that he included in the science of osteopathy (*Contributions of Thought - The Collected Writings of William Garner Sutherland, D.O.*, 1971, 293).

If you were on the ocean in a little barque and the waves were rolling high upon the shore, you would bring in the tension on the fulcrum in accordance with the balance point. In a spiritual intelligence, a spiritual fulcrum, you would be carried by the Tide in your little barque. You can depend on the Intelligence of the Tide and the potency of this fluid, the fluctuation of this fluid (*Teachings in the Science of Osteopathy*, 1990, 14).

The fluctuation of the Tide is a movement coming in during inhalation and ebbing out during exhalation. Is it the waves that come rolling along the shore, is that the tide? No. The movement of the tide is the movement of that body of water, the ocean, that constant body of water. See that potency in the tide; more power, more potency in that tide than there is in the waves that come dashing upon the shore (*Teachings in the Science of Osteopathy*, 1990, 15).

You can depend on the Intelligence of the Tide and the potency of the fluid (*Teachings in the Science of Osteopathy*, 1990, 14).

It is the stillness of the Tide, not the stormy waves that bounce upon the shore, that has the potency, the power (*Teachings in the Science of Osteopathy*, 1990, 16).

Allow the physiological function within to manifest its own unerring potency rather than apply a blind force from without (*Teachings in the Science of Osteopathy*, 1990, xii).

Where is that cerebrospinal fluid? Is it only in my body? No. It is in each and every one of your bodies. There is an ocean of cerebrospinal fluid in this room. Here is a fluid within a fluid. There is a fluid within a fluid. The Breath of Life is within each (*Teachings in the Science of Osteopathy*, 1990, 169).

It is not the outflow so much as a change or transmutation in that fluid-something that goes out from that quiver-an invisible something, which you might call the nerve force, and it follows along out to the area where its terminals dwell with the lymphatics. A change in its constituents or elements, through a transmutation...Dr. Still in his vision, referred to it as 'the highest known element in the human body' (*Contributions of Thought - The Collected Writings of William Garner Sutherland, D.O*, 1971, 200-201).

We refer to the potent fluctuation of this Tide and to something that is intelligent, something invisible (*Teachings in the Science of Osteopathy* 1990, 32).

Within the cerebrospinal fluid there is an invisible element that I refer to as the 'Breath of Life.' I want you to visualize the Breath of Life as a fluid *within* this fluid, something that does not mix, something that has potency as the thing that makes it move (*Teachings in the Science of Osteopathy*, 1990, 14).

It was recognition of the supreme potency of the Breath of Life as the *initiative spark* to involuntary activity that interpreted my synthesis relative to the primary respiratory mechanism (*Contributions of Thought - The Collected Writings of William Garner Sutherland, D.O 1971, 142-143*).

You merely see the spark from the positive and negative poles – it jumps from one pole to the other. But you do not see the real element because you are the man formed from the earth and walking about utilizing this breath of air. If you recognized the real element, the *breath of light* in the fluctuation of the cerebrospinal fluid, I think you would begin to come closer to the success of Dr. Still in his knowledge of the human body (*Contributions of Thought - The Collected Writings of William Garner Sutherland, D.O., 1971, 290-291*).

I want you to see this invisible 'liquid light', or the Breath of Life (*Teachings in the Science of Osteopathy, 1990, 34*).

There is a positive pole and a negative pole. Then we get something in between the positive and the negative poles to see in that slow movement of the Tide, that coil, a moving out and a coming together. How many spiral movements can you visualize in the Tide?...Watch this seaweed moving rhythmically in a coiling form, one going clockwise, another counterclockwise, spiraling with the groundswell. Look at the hurricane. See the potency in the eye of the hurricane, not the destruction around the outside. See the potency of the eye, the stillness of the Tide, the spiral movement" (*Teachings in the Science of Osteopathy, 1990, 17*).

We are referring to the Breath of Life in that Tide (*Teachings in the Science of Osteopathy, 1990, 32*)

According to the authority of the scriptural record, the Breath of Life, not the breath of material air, was breathed into the nasals of a form of clay and man became a living soul. If this record may be considered as literally true, then it agrees with the synthesis of a primary respiratory mechanism - an involuntary mechanism that includes fundamentally that highest known element, the cerebrospinal fluid, within which dwells that invisible Breath of Life (*Contributions of Thought - The Collected Writings of William Garner Sutherland, D.O.,* 1971, 216).

The "Breath of Life" is the spark, primarily, and not the breath of *air*. The breath of air is merely one of the material elements that the Breath of Life utilizes in man's walkabout here on earth (*Contributions of Thought - The Collected Writings of William Garner Sutherland, D.O.,* 137).

"Be Still" these physical senses and get as close to your Maker as you can-closer than breathing. Where you realize what is meant by the Breath of Life, not the breath of air - the breath of air being merely one of the material substances which man utilizes in his walkabout on earth ... by *knowing,* I mean not information gained by physical senses but a knowledge that comes from getting as far as one can from the physical sense. (*Contributions of Thought - The Collected Writings of William Garner Sutherland* 209-210)

I think the greatest discoveries will be made along spiritual lines. Someday people will have learned that material things do not bring happiness and are of little use in making men and women creative and powerful. Then the scientists of the world will turn their laboratories over to the study of God and prayer and spiritual forces which as yet have been hardly touched or scratched. When that day comes the world will see more advancement in one generation than has been seen in the last generations (*Contributions of Thought,* 293-4).

Just for a moment, think of your body being formed from that glass. That you are a glass house through which this Breath of Life may be reflected. Not even touching your house, your glass house, but being reflected through and through. See that sun reflecting itself upon the moon and then see the reflection from the moon all through the ocean. Reflection that does not touch the ocean, but lights them up. Makes a beautiful picture. Light! Liquid Light! (*Contributions of Thought*, 298)

ADAH SUTHERLAND:

He (Dr. Sutherland) did not hesitate to go beyond the evidence of the senses, penetrate deeply, and draw abundantly from the integrity and realities of the unseen. Each day, and this was frequent, he turned to what he alluded to as "pause-rest" periods; periods of silence with no outward evidence of activity. This was done with utmost simplicity and natural-ness... He liked the phrase "listening to silence" and used as an analogy the composer who makes as powerful use of silences as he does of sounds - of "communicative silences." Two freshets upon which he drew for nourishment of inner resources were "Be still and know" and "Closer is He than breathing." When the period of teaching arrived, he referred to these on occasion with unaffected naturalness because they were an integral part of his philosophy and his daily living. Dr. Sutherland had no denominational affiliation but... he was affiliated (A. Sutherland, *With Thinking Fingers,* 1962, 32, 65-66).

ROLLIN BECKER

If we, as student are to understand, we will find it necessary to reawaken our knowledge of the Deity that centers us, make it our Spiritual Fulcrum for our guidance, and learn to think, feel, and use the Creator in our daily practices (*Life in Motion,* 1997, 24)

The Master Fulcrum might almost be compared to a Master Spiral for the total mechanism, with hundreds of smaller ones (spirals) for individual function (*The Stillness of Life*, 2000, 179).

The Breath of Life is the individual spark of *Light* that centers the individual...; the cause lies within the Light, the Fulcrum (*The Stillness of Life*, 2000, 187).

There is far more to the Master Fulcrum than can be described or told about. I am conscious of being in the presence of the factor that makes us tick. Knowledge of what I am working with has created a sense of something so tremendous that all my sense of values is going to have to be revised (*The Stillness of Life*, 2000, 179).

The Breath of Life, the spark, the still point between the hand of God reaching out to the creation of Adam, that is the spark that initiates the functioning of the primary respiratory mechanism (*The Stillness of Life*, 2000, 124)

In the transmutation process the Boss steps into the Fulcrum, there is a great deal more that goes on than a mere loss of a pattern of dysfunction... a Rebirth, Regeneration of physical, mental, and emotional structure." (*The Stillness of Life*, 2000, 212)

When you are dealing with the highest known energy that's available, it does not want anyone interfering with what it is trying to do (*Life in Motion*, 1990, 48).

There is an individualized pattern of health for each individual person on earth... that is established from conception (*Life in Motion*, 1997, 47-48).

Stillness, to me, is the very key to what Dr. Will [Sutherland] was trying to give us. He made statements like, 'allow physiologic function to manifest its own unerring potency rather than use blind force from without." He is talking about a dynamic, direct experience that is this stillness. It isn't what we call the still point; there are trillions of those. It is this stillness, which is the motive force in the concept I use in my clinical practice... I get my hands under a given area of problem and I try to be aware of stillness. Not a still point, but a stillness that is that individual. You can only be conscious of stillness; you cannot palpate stillness with your hands. The stillness is that which centers every molecule of being of that living body (*The Stillness of Life*, 66-68).

Your Silent Partner is a fulcrum point; it's absolutely still. There's no energy in motion in the Silent Partner, none. It's all energy, but it's not in motion. Actually, it is the source of energy, the state from which energy comes. It isn't energy in motion, it's just pure potency. It's omnipotent. There is no motion, and yet it's all motion. It just is, and you surrender to it (*The Stillness of Life, 2000*, 30).

There is a fundamental Potency or Power that exists within all things that is alive for as long as they are alive. All life springs forth from this power, and the nature of this power is stillness, a dynamic stillness full of potential (*Life in Motion*, 1997, xviii).

I discovered a very beautiful description of the stillness written by another eastern philosopher. This man was listening to an artist playing a very complicated Indian musical instrument...Suddenly the watcher, the listener, disappeared; he had not been lulled into abeyance by the melodious strings, but was totally absent. There was only the vast space which is the mind. All of the things of the earth and of man were in it, but they were at the extreme outer edges, dim and far off. Within the space where nothing was, there was a movement, and the movement was stillness. It was a deep, vast movement, without direction, without motive, which began from the outer edges, and with incredible strength was coming towards the center-a center that is everywhere within the stillness, within the motion which is space. This center is total aloneness, uncontaminated, unknowable, a solitude which is not isolation, which has no end and no beginning. It is complete in itself, and not made; the outer edges are in it but not of it. It is there, but not within the scope of man's mind. It is the whole, the totality, but not approachable (*The Stillness of Life*, 2000, 68).

This is the stillness of the Tide...the stillness found at the fulcrum point within the Tide. There is a Potency *within* this stillness (*Life in Motion*, 1997, 29-30).

So, we are discussing something that occurs in a *vital mechanism in a time sequence* when all the factors that lead to its appearance are properly tuned for it to happen. Does this stillness have an inert feeling of lifelessness or absence of vitality? No. It is a living thing that has the feeling of power and Potency within it. It cannot be explained for I have no words to describe it, but it does happen and it is beneficent (*Life in Motion*, 1997, 30).

The cerebrospinal fluid has a Potency within it, a Breath of Life principle, a Highest Known Element-a fluid within a fluid. This invisible factor is found at the midway point between inhalation and exhalation, a fulcrum point in the tidal shifting...This Potency is found at the point of balance for the cerebrospinal fluid tide (*Life in Motion*, 1997, 95).

PAUL LEE

The love of God is present everywhere, preexisting, generating and permeating everything. Our physical forms exist in this sea, differentiating from it only by having managed to reduce the vibration of its material constituents as they manifest (*Interface: Mechanisms of Spirit in Osteopathy*, 2005, 155).

He (Dr. Sutherland) believed that this subtle inherent motion in the tissues was an exposition of spirit, another word for his breath of life. For Still, the life force or Unconditional Love is the very ground substance of all creation (*Interface: Mechanisms of Spirit in Osteopathy*, 2005, 255).

The indication of the two, spirit and matter creates form and motion, the two requirements of life. This interaction, according to Still, involves a reciprocal activity between the Celestial and the Terrestrial realms. In a similar respect, Dante said, "The Love of God, unutterable and perfect, flows into a pure soul the way that light rushes into a transparent object." This image of a substance flowing from God into humans is similar to the models expressed by Swedenborg and Still. The image created by these three men, Dante, Swedenborg, and Still is one of a sea of energy (love of God) from which the living form is created and in which it continues to exist, and by which it is nourished (*Interface: Mechanisms of Spirit in Osteopathy*, 77-78).

The embryo acquires space from the surrounding fluid medium in order to grow rather than growing solely by the process of cellular multiplication and expansion from within. At the end of a limb bud, for example, the embryo first establishes influence over the space into which it will grow within the fluid medium. Then it sends its multiplying cells into the appropriated space. The form is first created in fluid; the material body follows (*Interface: Mechanisms of Spirit in Osteopathy*, 112).

JACQUES ANDREVA DUVAL

"Four components are necessary as a practitioner, but they are acquired slowly through a process of initiation, total surrender, and years of practice and devotion:

The ability to be in stillness.

To possess a relationship with the 'silent partner.'

Have awareness of the fulcrum of light.

Possess the ability to be totally open or 'surrendered.'

A fulcrum is a relationship in which the Osteopath must do nothing, save to become one with the patient. The only work for the practitioner is the transformation of the self; that is, the Osteopath himself. In other words, the Osteopath's own spiritual growth. What you have to change, to transform totally, it is you, and you only. Understand?" (*Techniques Ostoépathiques d'Équilibre et d'Échanges Réciproques: Introduction à l'approche ostéopathique du Dr. Rollin Becker, DO, 122*)

ROBERT FULFORD

The cerebrospinal fluid seems to act as a storage field and a conveyor for the stepped down current from the sound and light energies. These fine essences of energy traverse up and down in the central canal of the spinal cord and are conducted by the fluid media of the spinal canal through all the fine nerve fibers in the body. They are related to the respiratory function and the manifestation of life in the body (Cisler, *Are We On The Path? The Collected Works of Robert C. Fulford*, 2003, 102- 103).

"The Light of Spirit projects outward as two sexed light waves (electric current). The light waves are made up of two polarities, positive polarity and negative polarity; thus, creating an interplay between the polarities at the neutral point or rod" (Cisler, *Are We On The Path? The Collected Works of Robert C. Fulford*, 143).

STEVE PAULUS

We must maintain a conscious engagement with the Stillness manifested in a Fulcrum during our work as Osteopaths. Ultimately, it doesn't matter how we interpret or name the forces of

Nature that do the work of healing. We only need to maintain our conscious spiritual connection via the "Wire" of continuity. Having a conscious spiritual connection was, I believe, the essence of "Dr. Still could not speak of." What he could not speak of is our true reference point as Osteopaths (Steve Paulus, *The Osteopathic Experience of Fulcrums and the Emergence of Stillness*, 2006, 200).

FRITZ SMITH

The vibrations of our auric fields affect our surroundings through the principle of resonance...As people come together their auric fields engage. There may be an instant sense of 'connecting' or 'bonding as both persons' inner 'tuning forks' of energy resonate at the same pitch...Resonance is facilitated if there is a shared experience or physical contact. The rituals of shaking hands, hugging or making other salutary greetings are ways of lessening the tension and implementing resonance between the two fields... like notes struck on a musical instrument to make a chord, as they move toward synchronization or harmony... as the current of energy flows through the spine and around the spinal bends, as I believe it does, vortices of energy would be created at the major curves. As I studied the skeleton and imagined these vortices whirling, I recalled a picture of a meditating yogi with the overlay of the spinal chakras, and instinctively knew that the chakras must exist. They were not just abstract symbols of an ancient religious system; they actually corresponded to the structure of the human skeletal system and the laws of physics (*Inner Bridges*, 1990, 42-42, 49).

WALTER RUSSEL'S INFLUENCE ON DRS. STILL, SUTHERLAND, AND BECKER

Walter Russell, the philosopher, scientist, and mystic, was a friend and teacher of Dr. Sutherland and Dr. Becker. Walter Russell expanded the meaning of the living fulcrum as, "the principle of equal giving between all moving pairs of unbalanced opposites, which constitute the dual electric universe... Rhythmic balanced interchange is the inviolate law, which must be obeyed." (*The Secret of Light*, 1947, 107).

Russell's book the *Divine Iliad*, characterizes the fulcrum as an inviolate law of balance: "I have but one law for all my opposed pairs of creating things; and that law needs but one word to spell it out, so hear me when I say that the one word of My law is BALANCE. And if man needs two words to aid him in his knowing of the workings of that law, those words are BALANCED INTERCHANGE. If man still needs more words to aid his knowing of my one law, give to him another one, and let those three words be RHYTHMIC BALANCED INTER-CHANGE." (*The Message of the Divine Iliad, Vol. 1 & 2* 1971, 74-75).

Russell then extended the fulcrum into the spiritual domain as, "A lever, moving upon its fulcrum expresses the idea of power by motion, but the power is in the *still fulcrum*. Power is not in the moving lever... all motion is a two-way extension of stillness... Everything in nature is a moving extension from the Stillness of the One Magnetic Light of God... Light and Stillness alone holds the potential energy for the expression of pattern. These two opposite unbalanced conditions violently desire to return to the oneness of balance from which they were divided into two. When the tensions cease, the conditions set up by them cease. Waves express the idea of the power of the ocean, but the power and the idea are in the calm of the ocean whether expressed by waves or not. The turbulence of the ocean springs from its calm, just as the movement of the lever springs from its still fulcrum" (*The Secret of Light*, 1947, 16, 39, 120, 139-140, 197-198)

Note: After Dr. Sutherland moved to Pacific Grove, California, he named his house The Fulcrum.

POTENCY AS A DESIRE FOR UNION

"Potency is the desire expressed by two opposing waves of light to return to oneness. The outstanding characteristic of waves is that they forever interchange. So long as equality of interchange continues rhythmically, waves repeat their interchange... credits and debits are balanced... they cease to be. They do not become one... opposites thus cancel each other out by interchange... they do not neutralize each other, as commonly believed - they cease to be... they become voided *and another thing from which both are extended, appears in their place.*" The above explains how the underlying pattern of health emerges out of stillness. (*The Secret of Light*, 1947, 107)

THE CADUCEUS REVISITED

One pole pulls inward spirally from within against its opposing pole, which thrusts outward spirally from within. This two-way radial universe of seeming motion is the product of these two opposed electric conditioners of matter which pass through each other in opposite directions. Each pole interchanges with the other in sequential pulsations as they pass through each other from points of gravity to wave field boundaries and back again in endless cycles. Each becomes the other at halfway rest points of their cycles.... The centering for every mass is still magnetic Light. Likewise, the still axis of every vortex is still magnetic Light... The one centering axis of both spirals is the shaft upon which the dynamic universe rotates. All motion rotates and revolves upon still centering shafts, and all shafts are two-way extensions of points which lead to and through centers of spheres... Wave pistons of light, or of the ocean, operate radially and spirally inward and outward, toward and away from gravity"...the still axis of every vortex is still magnetic Light (*The Secret of Light*, 1947,108, 128, 136, 148, 169 228, 249).

THE FULCRUM OF THE HUMAN BEING

God is the fulcrum of man, and of the universe... Man is a stepped down crystallization of Universal Light created by gravitational forces and expressed as an equilibrium between opposing spirals." (*The Secret of Light*, 1947, 115).

The imagined universe of My dual thinking is a two-way inter-changing between unbalanced lever ends of light, which extend from Me, their fulcrum of power in Rest, and return to Me. Behold in Me the fulcrum of my changing universe which manifests change, though I change not, nor move. For I am Rest. In Me alone is Balance. He who would find power must know that he extends from Me, that I am he. He who would find rest must return to Me, be Me, be the fulcrum of his own power (*The Secret of Light*, 1947, 172).

EMANUEL SWEDENBORG: HIS INFLUENCE ON DRS. STILL AND SUTHERLAND

Emanuel Swedenborg, anatomist, physiologist, mystic, and philosopher influenced both Dr. A. T. Still and Sutherland's osteopathic principles. Swedenborg was the first scientist to record the fluctuant circulation patterns of the CSF. He also postulated a step-down model by which the human being is created, stating that, "all things are related... in succession, from the infinite to the grossest level of the natural world" (Bell, 2006, 8).

Swedenborg's ascending categories from the human to the Divine include:

DIVINE ⇨ SPIRITUAL ⇨ CELESTIAL ⇨ VORTICAL ⇨ SPIRAL ⇨ SPHERE ⇨ ANGULAR

Swedenborg asserts that each level in the descent from spirit to matter contains all the levels which precede it, "the *vortical* form determines and enters into the *spiral*, and by the mediation of the *spiral*, the *sphere/circular*, and again by the mediation of the *circular*, the *angular*, all of which is within the *voritcal* form, not actually, but potentially" (Swedenborg, *Economy of the Animal Kingdom, III The Fibre* 1918, 184).

External form is born after the image of internal form, but not the reverse. For if from an *angular* form, the angles are cut off and the planes rounded, the form is turned into the *spherical*, or more perfect; but the internal form still remains (Swedenborg, *Economy of the Animal Kingdom, III The Fibre*, 1918, 174).

The *angular* is, "unsuited to the continuation of motion... The verimost form of motion... is the *spiral*. For its determinations are not into continuous concentric circles, nor are they directed by means of radii or straight lines to any common center; but they strive by means of continual spirals *to flow towards* a certain middle circle, occupying the place of a center that is void of angles and planes ... instead of lines we substitute forces, all the forces have regard to one single center wherein they all meet together in every possible relation of opposition... The *spiral* form is "a fluxion once commenced is continued with so easy a potency as to be almost spontaneous; and that nature has inscribed this faculty, potency, and force into the spiral flux is clearly apparent from the helix and screw in mechanics" (Swedenborg, *Economy of the Animal Kingdom, III The Fibre* 1918, 172-177, 180, 182).

SWEDENBORG'S VORTICAL FORM IS SUTHERLAND'S AUTOMATIC SHIFTING FULCRUM

Swedenborg refers to the *vortical* as a, *"Perpetuo-spiral,* or the *spiral* that is in constant motion... able to gyrate around its center, and can gyrate around as many centers as there are points in the periphery of the circle to which it has respect... there is not the least trace of opposition, but a certain natural spontaneity... the idea of the *vortical* form almost transcends the human understanding because it transcends geometry and its lines and curves... For into this *vortex* flow the parts and volumes of the *superior ether*, which constitute the great vortex around our earth... which are due to the marvelous iron-attracting faculty of the magnetic forces, besides many other phenomena occurring around the magnet. For it is an evident truth that such a form can in no way exist by the fluxion of substances of this nature, unless poles be assigned to it, and greater and lesser circles, just as in the great *sphere*; so that in any *vortical* form, least or greatest, there necessarily exists a certain pole, Arctic and Antarctic, with the idea of an axis and moreover, an equator (Swedenborg, *Economy of the Animal Kingdom* 1918, 185-187).

Transcending the *Vortical* form are three levels of spirit that Swedenborg named and ordered as the *Celestial, Spiritual* and *Divine.* "...the *Celestial* form enters into and determines the *vortical*... that which receives forms of all kinds should be itself void of all form...an invisible form void of figure and yet capable of figures... flows the universe called heaven, that is, each solar or stellar vortex... The *Spiritual* form receives the *Divine*, which is "not properly a form, but pure essence, life, intelligence, wisdom, and most utterly abstracted from space, time, matter, figure, motion, change, destruction" (*Economy of the Animal Kingdom, III The Fibre*, 1918, 188, 191-192, 194).

FROM EMPTINESS TO FORM THAT RETURNS TO EMPTINESS

"These forms are created for and accommodated to, not only the beginning of motion, but also the reception of life and intelligence by means of influx from the *Spiritual* form." He points out that form is created for the purpose of reception of *Spirit*. In naming seven rungs on the ladder of ascension, Swedenborg places the *vortex* as the midpoint or fulcrum between spirit and man. (*Economy of the Animal Kingdom, III The Fibre*, 1918, 196)

Swedenborg said the cerebrospinal fluid CSF has a spiral motion: "...the cortical gland, in respiring, expelling fluid, and producing fiber, makes spiral gyres. The CSF, which courses through this fiber,...seems to wind itself, both as to parts and as to volume, into the form of a similar gyre... As now regards the form of fluxion of the simple fiber, which produces the tensile of the aforementioned compound fiber, this form cannot be simply a *spiral* but must be superior to the spiral. For as forces and substances are elevated by degrees, so they are elevated into a superior and more perfect nature and potency. So, likewise with this form of fluxion, which therefore merits to be styled the *perpetuo-spiral*...we will call the *Vortical* (*Economy of the Animal Kingdom, III The Fibre*, 1918, 170).

THE SACRED TREMOR AND ENTRAINMENT

Swedenborg says that *tremulation* is the vibratory nature of motion, a fulcrum "permeating all the space of the Infinite universe" (Schooley, *The Fulcrum. 1953 OCA* Journal, 31). The *tremulation* of a string will cause a sympathetic vibration in another string; a membrane similarly affects another membrane; that is, if both are tuned in the same key. If the string of a lute is touched, it will cause a vibration in the other strings which are tuned in the same key... much of our vital force consists in tremulations. From the above rules it can be shown that our mobile life, or our nature, consists in little vibrations, that is, tremulations. A most minute particle is able to communicate its motion to all other things in the whole body, is able to bring a certain membrane and sinew, the blood, the life, and the spirit into the same motion with itself, and thereby all contiguous membranes, fibers, and nerves... It also frequently happens that a person falls into the thought of another person, that he perceives what another is doing and thinking, that is, that his membrane trembles from the tremulation of the other person's cerebral membranes, just as one string is affected by another, if they are tuned in the same key" (Swedenborg, *On Tremulation*, 1899, 2-6).

MODERN SPIRITUAL TEACHERS

Rudolf Steiner: The Direction of Your Heart's Breath Connects You With God, or to the Ego

Here I paraphrase Rudolf Steiner's characterization of the realizations when the whole body is an organ of perception, "we must learn to sense with the whole body as a sense of touch. In the head, if we let awareness recede behind the thought, into the brain core, and from there, allow our everyday thinking to relax, then our perception will expand past the horizon to infinity where it rests in stillness. When our own thoughts become still, thinking becomes a cosmic activity that originates from beyond the body. This new thinking from the beyond is perceived as an activity of light, which weaves the archetypal pictures that are the original ideas of form that weave as waves in the world like a refined breathing of light."

If this breathing focuses in on the self (ego), then personal thought forms develop into finished concepts and self-contained ideas. If you let your thinking freely expand and continue in waves, then cosmic ideas of movement arise in the heart. One perceives this as the movement of life that comes from the periphery. In the heart is the feeling, yet when a feeling is sensed into while one becomes quiet and still, one begins to sense the cosmic life that arises out of the heart's feelings. Then feeling becomes the Breath of Life. The fluids are both the source for the formation of the body and the touchstone for the ether, which contains the forces of the Breath of Life of the cosmos. This Breath of Life, connected to water, is the substance of cosmic forming. When sensed, it is a very blissful feeling as the sense of warmth that moves as life in the world; this warmth gives us our sense of humanity.

On a deeper level, even though breathing is the process of the lungs and the blood coursing downward into the body, inner breath also rises upward from the heart as light, vibration, and tone that expands in the brain and throughout the senses. When we breathe in, we receive the life of being of the spiritual world, and when we breathe out, our being flows out into the world. Here go the waves of breathing, rising to the brain core, into the light, and the waves light up. Light is everything that worked inwardly through the senses - hearing, seeing, taste, touch, smell - all are breath upon which light is weaving, waving, surging like the sunlight on the ocean sparkling through the waves. Willing rises to the head and becomes thought, and thought descends to become will.

As it descends to the limbs as light, thought becomes a subtle will activity. Willing is the movement of air, the all-pervading cosmic life, and in the instant that we open to this, our separate self disappears. This is known as the descending current, a reversal of the kundalini that takes place after one has opened awareness beyond the ego, and connected with that which is beyond it. (*The First Class Lessons and Mantras*)

Neil Cohen

I await even your slightest movements toward the feeling heart so I may come into expression and give you the gift of your Self - the Awakened Radiance of Love, Wisdom, and Intimacy. Fear, stress, tension, and anxiety is that portion of your being which has not yet relaxed into the fearless union of feeling and knowing the True Self, the Heart, the Origin of Being. (*Voice of Heart*, 2004, Self Published. 6)

Carl Jung

Purusha, the archetypal man is realized at Anahata (in the heart). Here is an experience of the essence of man, the supreme man, and the so-called primordial man. This is the first inkling of a within of your psychological or psychic existence that is not yourself, in which you are contained, which is greater and more important than you, but which has an entirely psychical existence. If you function in your Self, you are not your self - that is what you feel. You have to do it (life) as if you were a stranger, your life becomes an objective life not your own, but the life of a greater one, the Purusha. 'It is not I that lives, it is Christ that liveth in me.' (*The Psychology of Kundalini Yoga*, 40-47, 69)

Neil Douglass-Klotz

Sophia is when you make the two one, and when you make the inner as the outer, and the outer as the inner, and the above the below...then, you enter the kingdom. There must be this change of your orientation inwardly toward the heart. By turning inward to sense from outer to inner, you sense toward the inside rather than the outside, and you follow body awareness back to its source. This new sensing, the sacred sense, is the

Sophia, the Holy Wisdom. It is a Breath of individuality that arises from a sense of innerness, which expands to connect with the Sacred Unity to form the original, integrated I AM, the Self (*The Hidden Gospel.* 30).

Sri Aurobindo

"The heart and the whole being may respond to the secret divine Ananda and change itself into this true original essence. Faith and will must be accompanied by and open into an illimitable widest and most intense capacity for love... the main business of the heart, its true function is love... This is the highest and the most characteristic perfection of the heart." (*The Highest Perfection of the Heart* - From *The Synthesis of Yoga* (1990) Lotus Press).

"According to the ancient teaching the seat of the immanent Divine, the hidden Purusha, is in the mystic heart - the secret heart-cave, hrdaye guhayam, as the Upanishads put it, and, according to the experience of many Yogins, it is from its depths that there comes the voice or the breath of the inner oracle." (*The Path of the Heart for Spiritual Realization* - From *The Synthesis of Yoga* (1990) Lotus Press).

APPENDIX 4
STUDY GUIDE

The following experiential realizations were crafted in mutuality by students during a Woodacre, CA *Mentor Course* in 2006 to help them attune to and distinguish the subtle inner body breaths *as* expressions of consciousness.[64]

THE CRANIAL WAVE IS NERVOUS SYSTEM MOTION

The cranial wave rate varies based on the amount of stress that is present; it is not the steady whole-body tidal ebb and flow of primary respiration. Cranial wave stillpoints are local events in the tissues; whereas after stillness pervades the whole-body, the cranial wave disappears and is replaced by primary respiration. Fluid flow consciousness is prior-to, and thus, beyond the cranial wave and the nervous system's capacities. The qualities of the cranial wave nervous system motion also vary because it reflects the many ways that consciousness recoils when it is trapped by narcissistic ego-driven control strategies that create separation from love. Below are the many qualities of the cranial wave reported by *Stillness Touch* practitioners:

- I feel a buzz inside my body.
- There is a slight tremor in my hands.
- I am hyper-alert.
- My mind moves fast with rapid staccato, spinning thoughts.
- I am aware of inner-body static.
- I feel vigilant.
- I am slightly paranoid.
- I have strong emotions of doubt, mistrust, suspicion, rage, hatred.
- I am not OK with what is, or how others are.
- I feel irritation, impatience, lack of compassion, and a tendency to complain because I feel angry because what is happening is not my way.
- I regularly check if my environment is safe or not.
- My breath is shallow and I may be breathing as rapid as every second.
- With my eyes closed my self-reflective consciousness and my body disappears, I lose myself, and since there is no container I feel anxiety.
- I have a fast-paced, head oriented thinking, a grasping ego, and low-grade panic. My thoughts race and cascade static-like, which tightens my muscles and creates body armor in my jaw, solar plexus, and perineum that are chronically tight. I have cold or numb hands and feet.
- I feel tortured by self-judgment and regularly search for wrongs in myself, in clients, and in others, and I want to fix them to gain self-value.
- I am in a task-oriented accomplish mode that is aimed at external results.
- I objectify and externalize my body, self, clients, others, and events.

- Neutral is another name for the natural state, which is a disposition, or attitude toward self and your recipient that is free from efferent activity. Neutral occurs by orienting within amid a quiet surrender of attention in which you sense and witness self-transformation directly.
- It is a letting be while orienting attention inward, leaving your inner process and the client's process *as it is*, while opening to the inherent radiance in the heart.
- This attitude of relaxed openness frees your fixed attention, and liberates the inertial energy that imprisons perception.
- As an anti-neutral act, efferent activity occurs when we leave our inner body space to objectify and separate the client into anatomical parts in order to evaluate the anatomy and then apply techniques, intentions, suggestions, visualizations, hold an agenda - even subtle ones such as loving-kindness, or loving suggestions, etc.
- Note: a biodynamic neutral begins as a whole-body stillness, whereas the cranial wave neutral is a local stillpoint in the tissues, which is not a biodynamic phenomenon.

COMPARING AN EFFERENT PRACTICE WITH STILLNESS TOUCH

An Efferent Practice

As your client walks in the door, you view their separate anatomical parts to determine how unbalanced and dis-eased they are and what needs fixing. You observe from a structure-function point of view, and you make contacts that help correct structural imbalances. Efferent activity is an outer directness of attention that automatically objectifies the client that turns them into a separate other. Efference also separates the recipient's body into anatomical parts to fix, treat, or heal by applying intentions, suggestions, naming tides, using focused perception, or even holding an attitude toward a client such as loving-kindness. Efference includes entering the recipient's body to feel their anatomy and seek out lesion patterns in the nervous system and using techniques to correct them; this is a very compelling lure of the medical model functional approach to cranial.

Stillness Touch Practice

You sense the recipient enter your session room as a whole human being as one unit. Given that you are not the doer who treats during a session, you wait in unknowing. If waiting is sincere, the potency *inside you* guides your attention, which synchronizes with the motion of health that arises as primary respiration. Primary respiration is in charge of your hand contacts, which as fulcra of stillness connect to the stillness in the recipient *without your help.* Your neutral touch reharmonizes the functions that, in turn, balance the tissues inherently. There is no doing to the recipient in any way; only a reposing within stillness.

HOW DOES A PRACTITIONER NEUTRAL BODILY FEEL TO A RECIPIENT?

When receiving a *Stillness Touch* session, you experience a distinct sense of the *presence of stillness.* Out of this stillness, subtle inner body breaths ebb and flow that rebalance areas of your body all by itself. You are only vaguely aware of the practitioner's personality, if at all. Sometimes you have to look to see if the practitioner is touching you because they are so out of the way. When areas that have been traumatized and contain shock are touched by primary respiration, you are able to both fully participate and witness the shock leave your body; when before, you were unable to be with the discomfort when a trauma was released.

WHAT IS YOUR EXPERIENCE WHEN A PRACTITIONER IS EFFERENT?

Your perception is forced to focus on the parts of your body with no ability to sense the whole body, which can lead to YOU disappearing into dissociation. Several possibilities occur when you leave your body: you become invisible, you may feel boredom during the session, you lack confidence in and distrust the practitioner, you may shut down, feel lost, and trapped. You can also feel suppressed by the force of the inertia that is in your anatomical parts, rather than feeling buoyantly held in the oneness of your whole-body breathing field. This suppression may continue as a feeling that your awareness is a prisoner to your traumas, rather than feeling your trauma release. The session can feel stressful rather than healing. Afterwards, you may feel chaotic and frantic because something was forced on you. You may rationalize why you allowed this to go on during the session, and you did not speak up, realizing once again, that leaving yourself behind reimburses the familiar feelings of self-betrayal, guilt, hatred, and shame. Basically, your system is over-whelmed because the practitioner controlled the session, ran energy into you, or used intention to force something to happen in the anatomy; rather than allowing a greater unerring force to do its work. After the session you may experience unclear muddled thinking, disorientation, anxiety, fatigue, dizziness, nausea, or low grade panic.

THE FIVE ENFOLDMENTS OF CONSCIOUSNESS: NERVOUS SYSTEM MOTION, FLUID FLOW, SPACIOUS LUMINOSITY, THE INFINITE BLACK PRESENCE OF STILLNESS, AND PURE BREATH OF LOVE

The purpose of this section is to support a practitioner in attuning to the inner body's tidal enfoldments. This is presented to enhance perception of yourself as you orient attention within your body space, and it creates a context for the recognition and deepening of your development of the natural state in each unfoldment.

Included for Each enfoldment:

1. General description, definition, or function.
2. The practitioner's experience.
3. Experience of being on the table.
4. What your whole-body-felt sense reveals, and the nature of the self that is experiencing itself unfolding into deeper states of wholeness.

WHEN NERVOUS SYSTEM MOTION SHIFTS TO FLUID FLOW

The felt-qualities of the cranial wave include rapid automatic repetition, variable tempos, electrically charged, digital, static, buzzing, shuttling, two-dimensional, and mechanical motion. Whereas in fluid flow the inner body-felt sense is of a slower, smoother, spontaneous expression of multidimensional, fractal, micromotion. The cranial wave disappears in whole body stillness out of which the steady ebb and flow of primary respiration arises.

- Your hands soften, and your touch feels buoyant, while

the heart expands, and since thoughts have less grip the inner anxiety and pressure relaxes and body tension decreases.

- Perception widens to the whole body, parts disappear, focus softens, and a subtle *breath* fills the whole body, thinking is less automatic and thoughts are slower; sensation is intensified yet, less defined, more diffuse, and less sharp, more porous.
- Your experiencing self shifts from objectively viewing your body as an object to an immersion in the body as subject.
- Once your awareness is inside the body, self becomes one with the body and its expressions.
- Breathing slows as it ascends and descends from the heart to deep into the belly and pelvis with an awareness of a subtler *breath* that breathes throughout the whole body (whole-body breathing).

FLUID FLOW: THE SOPHIA - THE SOUL REUNITES WITH THE BODY

Function of Fluid Flow in the Body

- Establishes healthy physiological functioning.
- Opens the midline and frees the subtle inner *breaths* that distribute to the body.
- Collects the separated body parts and unites them with the whole - all the way into the ground substance and cells, which optimizes function.
- Connects the inner and outer fields as one.
- You realize that whole-body felt sense is heart perception.
- Heart as an organ of perception unites thinking with your body-felt sense.

- The mind-body split reunites as bodymind.
- Personal perception reunites with nature; one perceives that the wisdom of the body and nature's wisdom are one.
- You recognize the arrival of your natural state.

Your Natural State in Fluid Flow

- The tempo of your inner sensing slows, awareness falls back into the body effortlessly, you come out of a sense of segmental anatomical body parts and enter a sense of the totality of the body as a unit - *this is the natural state.*
- Solid separate body parts liquify, and unify - the quality of the movement is sensed as a whole-body flowing, streaming, fluid sensation.
- Stillness fills your whole body and extends around the body from which a subtle inner body breathing arises.
- You open to a whole body sensing, that is at first more solid, and then becomes fluid as your awareness shifts to fluid flow.
- Potency is at first felt as a buildup of tension, vibration, or intensity that gives way and opens to pleasure, streaming, and an elegant fluid flow. Your hands shift from feeling like tissues, muscles, and bones, that become soft, porous, buoyant, fluid hands.
- Your poignant heart perceives as a whole-body felt-sense that expands to the field around your body and includes the one you touch.
- Thinking, feeling, and will harmonize and unify.
- Your body-felt sensing is brighter than thinking, but from the perspective of thinking it seems fuzzy.
- Your attention moves with primary breath: during Inspiration there is an intensification of poignancy, and in Expiration the poignancy recedes.

- You sense an intensification of the feeling tones within your whole-body during Inspiration, and then an ebbing of intensity during Expiration, in a steady 12-seconds for each cycle in synchrony with primary breath.
- Your subtle whole-body breath ascends and descends the midline in 12 second cycles in synchrony with primary respiration.
- You sense inner-body widening side to side/front to back during Inspiration, and a sense of centering and lengthening along midline during Expiration.
- Thoughts float freely, and there is a lessening of the ego griping, recoiling, or co-opting awareness.
- You feel in an intimate body-felt contact with the one you touch, and you are naturally entrained with them.
- You realize intimacy as a felt-sense of the *two in one*: one breath breathes the two of you.

Sense of Fluid Flow While You are on the Table

- You realize a perceivable shift from rapid, discreet, disjointed motions of the parts in the body to a unified whole-body flow.
- A felt-sense of an open heart from which you, as recipient, feel poignantly touched by and in intimate contact with the one touching you.
- Thoughts are resting, softly floating, and quiet.
- Breath is open and freely moves from chest to belly to pelvis.
- You sense contact with a mysterious presence that is wise, and which reveals the various aspects of the body moving in harmony as one unit, yet each portion moves to its own tune: this is the felt-sense of *coherent motion*.
- This same coherence is present in your thinking,

feeling, sensing, and will, which are all united and in synchrony; as opposed to each faculty functioning apart from one another and at war.

- There is a welling of intensification of enthusiasm, then a receding of intensity in synchrony with Inspiration and Expiration.
- Your previous sense of inner buzz, edginess, anxiety, irritation, inner pressure to know, vigilance, and paranoia is now sensed as ease, relaxation, flow, and a contentment with not knowing, along with a felt sense of trust in the inherent benevolence and wisdom of the process.
- Smooth, sensuous, and elegant motion feels intelligent in its flowing from place to place as though it is imbued with wisdom, while blocked places open up and join the breathing pond of the whole body that is moving *with* primary breath.
- All body parts disappear, and you sense the body as one whole unit that is intercommunicating, negotiating, harmonizing, and guided by 'something' that knows what it is doing; you sense wholeness and a connection to essence. This is the quality of the inherent wisdom of the body, the *Sophia,* or the Soul.
- You sense a center or midline that reconnects you to essence.
- Your sense of self is *inside* the body in touch with all its expressions, sensations, intelligence, and transmutations.
- Your perception is open, porous, soft, and boundaries fade, which may include contact with the subtle beings of nature such as plant beings, fairies, animal spirits, and other shamanic emanations.
- You have a whole-body felt sense of inner melting, warmth, tingling, dropping, sinking, opening, relaxing,

streaming, flowing, while tension of armor unfurls amid buoyancy that creates a sense of lengthening out of the bone sockets. There is a sensuous and erotically pleasurable flow in the body, yet not exclusively genitally focused.

- *Breath*: physical breath deepens in the body, drops to belly and pelvis; there can also be a feeling of heaviness and density in the body.
- *Awareness:* a natural concentration arises as the mind relaxes.
- The transition from fluid flow to luminosity occurs after stillness expands from the body into the room and to the edge of the known in which an extremely subtle breath of radiant presence arises.

SPACIOUS LUMINOSITY: THE TEMPLATE OF WHOLENESS

Function of Spacious Luminosity

- You can realize the *Self - I Am*.
- You realize the union between *Self* and Thou versus the prior sense of separation. between *self* as a me - not you.
- Your uncherished aspects feel accepted, seen, met, and loved unconditionally.
- Your natural state fructifies.

The Natural State Amid Spacious Luminosity

- When Stillness pervades the whole body, fills the room, and extends to the edge of your known to become unified consciousness, the self merges into the *Self* that connects you to 'the All' that then evolves you toward your life's destiny.

- Your soft, porous, fluid hands vaporize and become vast and luminous.
- Your heart field expands to the horizon of your known, or it spills over the edge of your known. Meanwhile, an infinitesimal point and the infinite periphery are united as one and you realize the *positionless position*.
- You sense a vast extremely subtle luminous breath that sees you as you are. Your personality structure and all your shadows feel seen, met, and held by an all-knowing *Presence* that loves us *as you are*. You feel self-love and unconditionally loved by a *Radiant Presence*.
- You may enjoy beatific encounters with archetypal emanations of the *Deity*: Buddha, Christ, Mary, Tara, Quan Yin, Eternal Feminine, Seraphim, Angels, Platonic Solids, and Luminous Geometric shapes and colors. Vibratory tones emanate the Template of Wholeness that creates the organizing fields of metabolic patterns in the subtle fluids, which create the functions that make the form - as the anatomy, to accommodate it.

Discerning Vast Luminosity on the Table

- A vast stillness fills your whole body, expands into the room, and extends to the edge of your known; meanwhile, a vast luminous breath suffuses the body from within and outside simultaneously.
- You sense a vast inner liquid light that breathes presence.
- You sense a delicate soft loving *Radiant Presence* that beholds you in unconditional love.
- You feel seen, met, held, and loved exactly *as you are*.
- The sense of love that you feel gives rise to an ardent desire to devote your life to this *Radiant Presence* to cultivate an irrevocable union with I Am That.

- There is an inner body-felt sense of vastness, shimmering, effervescence, and lightsome-ness.
- You enjoy Universal Consciousness *as* a spacious, vaporous luminescence that knows.
- You have extremely subtle perceptions of a tender, loving substance of Breath that builds the intensity of luminosity for nearly 1 minute, and then it recedes in the intensity for 1 minute.
- Your five separate senses unite into one sense with five facets while your whole body becomes an organ of perception - this is *Spiritual Touch* - by which you feel bodily in touch with everything.

DYNAMIC STILLNESS IS INFINITE BLACK SPACE

Your sense of *Self* builds in strength in the *Radiant Presence,* until at some point your consciousness expands into an infinite black stillness. Stillness engulfs the *Self,* and culminates in a total cessation: there is no sense of *Self,* time, space, or memory except in retrospect. Eventually with repeated contact, your presence remains awake inside Dynamic Stillness, which becomes your consciousness. This is the realization of I AM. There are no tides and the biodynamic map is gone.

Function of Dynamic Stillness

There is an instinctual felt-sense of Wholeness that defies description; you know healing has happened, yet you do not know how it occurred. Practically speaking, whether on the table or while touching there is nothing to do except "be still and know I AM." At this stage, there is only stillness - all motion ceases, including the breathing of primary respiration.

You have prepared yourself for this profound realization by your daily *Stillness Practice* that synchronizes your consciousness with Dynamic Stillness. Then, during your preparation before you touch the recipient, you inwardly orient awareness until your midline, your SA Node, and Dynamic Stillness become contiguous. You approach your recipient and touch them in and *as* neutral.

Dynamic Stillness *as* Your Natural state

- Your state changes when the luminous potency yields to infinite black Dynamic Stillness.
- Your heart expands beyond the horizon of your known to an unknowable infinity, and your awareness may return *as* Dynamic Stillness.
- Tidal rates are no longer relevant; you sense no rates, there is only Stillness.
- Dynamic Stillness is the absolute fulcrum that is realized at infinity, and your SA Node is your access to it because they are one.
- Your touch is with invisible hands of stillness.
- Healing simply *is*: there is no process, and no knowledge of what occurred until after the session is over.

Discerning Dynamic Stillness on the Table

All is still. You may discern increasing degrees of absorption of your consciousness in Dynamic Stillness, which at times can disappear. You are suspended in infinite black stillness that is all pervading. The sense of ordinary consciousness ceases, and in retrospect, it feels as though you have entered the 'nothing' and 'everything' at the same time. Be Still and Know.

Pure Breath of Love

Everything that occurs amid *Pure Breath of Love* is in mutuality: there is no meaningful distinction between the one offering touch and a recipient - there is no separation.

After the infinite black stillness implodes inside the body, there is no sense of distinct tides or separate states of consciousness. Your sense inside you is of a permanent seal of infinite black stillness in which pours a paradoxical substance that emanates *a whole-body pulse that is in tandem with the heartbeat.* This is *Pure Breath of Love.*

You realize that Dynamic Stillness is the unwavering foundation out of which all life arises and dissolves. When you pass "beyond" Dynamic Stillness, *Pure Breath of Love* emerges within. But this is not primary respiration, and it cannot be characterized as such because there are no tides, and no set rates that can be timed. You do sense rhythm - as ever-changing, multidimensional, polyrhythmic motions on all levels and depths at once, in the same moment, and in the same space - but it is not rational. You are in an undeniable direct contact with the Mystery of Life, which is self-evident to your whole-body felt sense.

This paradoxical state that is both extremely sublime and very dense, *Pure Breath of Love* feels like blazing mercury, or liquid dense lava that moves very slowly, and, at the same time, it expresses a billowing, nonphysical, nonliquid, non-potent "something" that is not anything, yet it bestows wholeness to every molecule in your body. This Wholeness-as-Health is ever-present, original, primordial, unborn, and it never dies. You know this, yet you cannot perceive how you know, and you do not care how or why you know because the truth is self-evident and, therefore, the mode by which this knowledge arrived is irrelevant. This is the quality of *Divine Ignorance.*

The potencies that accompany *Pure Breath of Love* can only be hinted at. They are at once sublime, soft, delicate, loving, strong, awesome, tough, ruthless, cutting, sweet, and tender. But, whatever the quality of the potency, you trust that it is whatever is needed, arises to reestablish seamless coherence throughout the whole-bodily being. Any attempt to describe this detracts from what it is. Contact with *Pure Breath of Love* is intimately connected to your destiny.

All to do as a practitioner is Be Still and Know.

GROUP DYNAMICS

How the Group Functions, Speaks, Moves, Operates.

When a group transitions from the cranial wave to fluid flow, instead of pinging off of each other and conversing in rapid staccato speech that is filled with the affects from the narcissistic personality structure, there is a whole group-sense of flow, a being with each other. Perceptually, in the fluid flow and vast luminosity everyone in the group feels connected during a touch demonstration: the one touching, the one being touched, and others in the room are all interconnected by the wisdom of the body, which is *united* with the wisdom of nature, and *Sophia* the wisdom of the world. At Dynamic Stillness, the need to talk and share experiences decreases dramatically; there is a group sense that everything that occurs is 'just so.' In the *Pure Breath of Love* the group sense of ordinariness deepens, which is due to an integration of all the prior states of consciousness. The group is content with not talking or sharing; rather the interest is in a deep repose in silence and savoring the depth of the group field.

APPENDIX 5
SELF-INQUIRY TO DEEPEN YOUR INNER-BODY AWARENESS

Be honest, and do not bypass this honest self- inquiry to *know thyself.*

Are you present inside your body? And do you recognize the qualities when you are present *inside* your body?

Catch if there is some part of your awareness that stays in your head and looks down into the body, rather than drowning inside the ocean of the inner body space.

Do you feel reposed in presence, regardless of what is going on inside or outside amid your daily activities? Being present usually results in a sense of inner repose regardless of what is happening.

A felt-sense of safety only occurs when we inhabit our body with presence.

Can you feel and then let go of specific tensions in your body without naming, trying to understand, or fixing them?

Are you reposed in a state of openness, rested in not knowing, not naming, and in innocence? And if you are not, can you be with that?

Are you perceiving spontaneously, or are you going after objects based on your prior experience by trying to visualize it to receive or get something? This the key to waiting, but not waiting *for* anything.

Can you be affected by what is inside you without defending, or recoiling?

Can you respond spontaneously to what is here with a fresh innocence?

In a *Stillness Touch* session, can you reflect on what happened after the session? Doing anything during the session is not neutral; it is an efferent activity.

How do you approach your experiences: is it with suspicion, trust, openness, doubt, fear, distancing, trying to understand, wanting to name or change them?

Are you intimate with your experience, or are you distancing by story-telling about it?

Can you let *what is* be *as it is* without it having to be different?

What is the felt-sense tonality of the elemental quality of your inner-body atmosphere? For example, is it a sense of Earth, Water, Fire, Air, Ether, or, are all the elements combined?

What Realm are you in, is it personal? Transpersonal? Ancestral? Universal? All and everything?

Is your perceptual field unconditional and beyond judgement?

Can your attention freely flow, or is it latched onto thoughts, experiences, speech, desires, and making meaning?

Can you allow changes in your states of consciousness and be with its resulting effects?

Can you not take away from, take care of, reassure, fix, change, name, or understand your experiences? Do you recognize that your inherent wisdom can navigate whatever comes up. When you can embody this practice, it resonates a confidence of being.

Can you allow an open field of free presence that is mildly curious, yet immersed in the innocence of not-knowing. In other words, you remain open, rather than closing your presence down too quickly by naming, drawing conclusions, making meaning, knee-jerk responses, habitual patterns of reactivity, and recoil.

While orienting inside, sense the qualities without naming. To distinguish between feelings, emotions, and sensation. Feelings and emotions are personal whereas sensations are universal. Sensing is direct and universal, whereas feelings and emotions are personal. For example, we all agree that a breeze flows along our skin; this is a universal sensation. Yet for some, the breeze will feel irritating, and for others it will feel soothing. The one who feels irritated may experience emotions, such as anger; while the one who feels soothed may have an emotion such as joy.

If you sense "nothing" can you characterize the qualities of nothing?

Can you stop meaning-making and simply become interested in what you are sensing right now"? This helps you stay present in the NOW.

APPENDIX 6
CHARTS

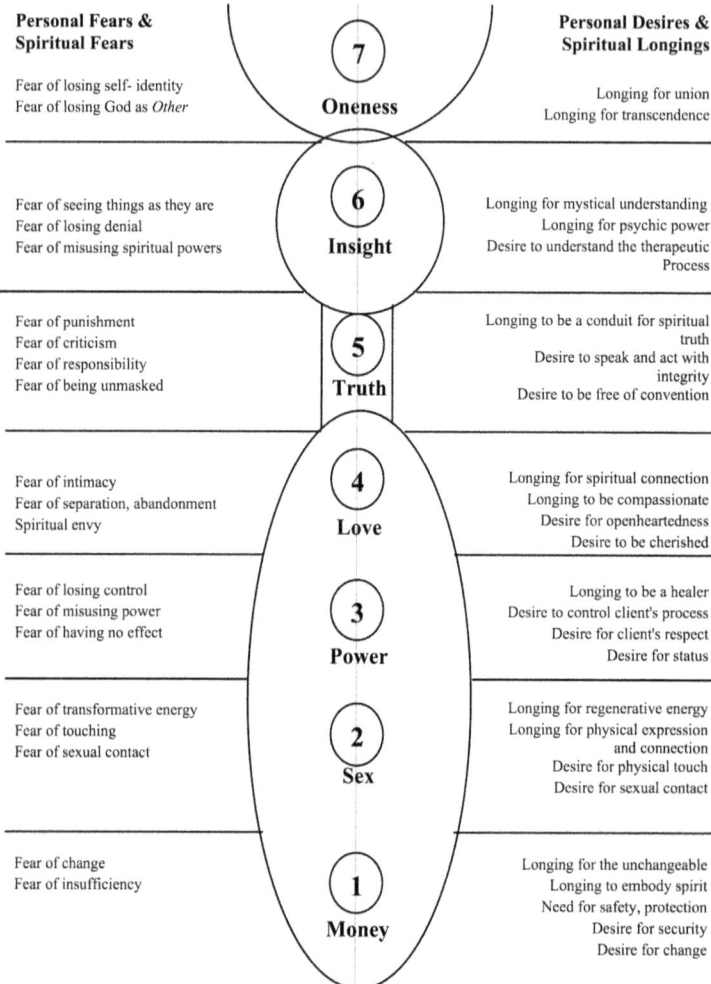

Personal Fears & Spiritual Fears		Personal Desires & Spiritual Longings
Fear of losing self- identity Fear of losing God as *Other*	**7** **Oneness**	Longing for union Longing for transcendence
Fear of seeing things as they are Fear of losing denial Fear of misusing spiritual powers	**6** **Insight**	Longing for mystical understanding Longing for psychic power Desire to understand the therapeutic Process
Fear of punishment Fear of criticism Fear of responsibility Fear of being unmasked	**5** **Truth**	Longing to be a conduit for spiritual truth Desire to speak and act with integrity Desire to be free of convention
Fear of intimacy Fear of separation, abandonment Spiritual envy	**4** **Love**	Longing for spiritual connection Longing to be compassionate Desire for openheartedness Desire to be cherished
Fear of losing control Fear of misusing power Fear of having no effect	**3** **Power**	Longing to be a healer Desire to control client's process Desire for client's respect Desire for status
Fear of transformative energy Fear of touching Fear of sexual contact	**2** **Sex**	Longing for regenerative energy Longing for physical expression and connection Desire for physical touch Desire for sexual contact
Fear of change Fear of insufficiency	**1** **Money**	Longing for the unchangeable Longing to embody spirit Need for safety, protection Desire for security Desire for change

Cargiver Vulnerabilities to Ethical Misconduct

Representation based on "Caregiver Vulnerabilites to Ethical Misconduct" by Kylea Taylor in "The Ethics of Caring: Honoring the Web of Life in our Professional Healing Relationships"

Charts Updated and Revised from the book STILLNESS				
Types of Cranial Work	**Biomechanical** *Pre-biodynamic*	**Functional** *Pre-biodynamic*	**Biodynamic** *Classic Biodynamic*	**Stillness Touch** *Post-biodynamic*
Degree of Efferent Application by the Practitioner (How much Doing is There?)	Cranial wave motility is not a guide, rather the cranial techniques require an extremely skilled application of precise physical forces to the cranial bones to create changes in the relationship between the sutures (*direct method*) or exaggerating the motion in its direction of ease (*indirect method*) to its endpoint and holding there until a stillpoint is induced, which affects a change in the tissues being treated, and function becomes more healthful.	The practitioner follows the cranial wave within its freedom of motion. In classical functional methods, there is no exaggeration of the motion, no holding at an endpoint, nor inducing a stillpoint. Local stillpoints arise naturally by waiting until the motion is inherently suspended and the tissues become buoyant - this is called a neutral. During neutral, the client's breath may be employed to assist in balancing the tissues, along with the autonomic nervous system balance, which combined affects the local stillpoint and creates physiological changes.	To realize a biodynamic neutral, a practitioner synchronizes with the motion present, fluid drive, potency, and primary respiration - all at once. She does not follow cranial wave or use the client's breath. She waits until the client is neutral after stillpoints in the local area spreads to stillness in the whole body. This is a neutral that begins a biodynamic session. Primary respiration - a delicate breathing field inside the client's whole body - suffuses potency in the fluids and tissues that transmutes inertial motion into coherent healthy fractal motion inherently throughout all systems.	There is zero efference or involvement. He is utterly surrendered to *Pure Breath of Love*, which is in total charge of the session. *Pure Breath of Love* addresses the needs of the client, by taking into account the entire spectral human being that includes their '*given*' - the history that is held in the tissues - and their infinitely evolving Spirit.
Therapeutic Forces the Practitioner Employs	Two methods are used: Direct method uses mechanical cranial techniques to move bones based on detailed knowledge of suture motion. With the Indirect method, one follows the motion of ease and exaggerates to an endpoint. Based on structure-function: Changes in structure creates functional change (direct), or function changes, and structure will rebalance (indirect method).	Support the permitted motion of the cranial wave until local stillpoint of neutral arises inherently, use the client's breath while a balanced autonomic nervous system creates a stillpoint that inherently arises and a dynamic exchange between the potency, fluids, and tissues ensues which will create a new function that affects changes in structure.	Synchronize with primary respiration - its potency creates the developmental motion that makes the fetus. After birth, primary respiration continues as an innate motion to maintain a healthy function in the body. Primary respiration creates potency in the fluids as a therapeutic force that segues to stillness in which primary respiration breathes healthy motion throughout the whole body.	No forces are applied on behalf of the practitioner. *Pure Breath of Love* does everything.

Breath	Cranial Wave	Fluid Tide	Long Tide	Dynamic Stillness	*Pure Breath of Love*
Rate or Motility	Variable rate: 7-14 cycles per minute Expands for approximately 4-6 seconds, and then recedes for approximately 4-6 seconds.	Steady rate: 2 ½ cycles per minute Expands for 12 seconds, then recedes for 12 seconds.	Invariable rate: 1 minute 40 second cycle: Expands for 50 seconds, then recedes 50 seconds.	No rate: Total cessation of all breaths.	*Pure Breath of Love* is a paradoxical state that consists of a precise combination of no rate, any rate, or all rates, which are within the one rate of the whole-body *Sacred Pulse* that is in tandem with the SA Node. This one rate emanates a super substance that is an alchemical mix that is specific to the client's needs. Depending on that need, one can perceive any rate that expresses in each enfoldment, as well as no rate of Dynamic Stillness. This is not logical, nor understandable; it simply is - as a characteristic of *Pure Breath of Love*.
Level of Human Consciousness	From Rational to Vision-logic. The domain of the Body-Mind Split	Psychic Body Mind Soul The Body- Mind split reunites.	Subtle *The Self*	Causal Pure Spirit	Non-dual and Beyond All levels of consciousness are present, ranging from the ego to the infinite as an utterly embodied suffusion of *Pure Breath of Love* into the inner space of each cell - all of which is ordinary. An infinite depth of wholeness is realized' there is no time, no space, no distance, no story, no unfolding. It is 'evolution' *as* the motion as it is in *Now*.

	Cranial Wave	Fluid Tide	Long Tide	Dynamic Stillness	*Pure Breath of Love*
Character of Each Level	The presence of cranial wave (CW) reflects the neurological functioning of the ego in modern life. Indigenous people have no cranial wave. CW rate changes are based on the client's status - whether they are calm, ill, stressed, injured, traumatized, etc. CW is a reactivity to the stressors of life. Like a vinyl record, the CW is a holographic record that reflects the client's past inertia, which is discerned by a practitioner who is skilled in reading the client's history in their tissues. In CW there are local stillpoints; CW disappears when a whole- body stillness arises as a biodynamic neutral.	The presence of primary respiration of fluid tide appears at a biodynamic neutral - when whole-body stillness arises. Primary respiration is sensed as a delicate whole-body breathing field that connects to the midline and reunites the recipient's body-mind split, and reorders the body's inertial motion patterns by transmuting them to healthy fractal motion. A practitioner's work is to Be *Still* as a neutral presence, while the inherent healing process engages its own sequence and order for wholeness. The practitioner includes in her awareness Primary Respiration, fluid drive, and motion present all at once.	The presence of primary respiration of long tide appears if a recipient's midline has re-balanced and there is a potent suffusion of global luminosity. Inertial patterns are reorganized by long tide en-mass, system-wide, on many levels at once. The recipient realizes the *Self*, and encounters archetypal exalted deities, sacred geometry, and tones. Perception shifts from the one who sees to feeling seen and contained by a *Radiant Presence* who beholds them in unconditional love - just as they are.	The *presence of stillness* only. An infinitely deep black stillness permeates every aspect of the recipient and practitioner. Healing occurs behind the curtain of awareness in a cloud of unknowing, yet there is a certainty that healing has occurred on a deep level. A sense of reverence is permanently instilled into consciousness, which eventually unites with stillness so deeply that there is no difference between Dynamic Stillness and your consciousness. I AM.	Pure Breath of Love is sealed inside Dynamic Stillness and contains all expressions of consciousness. The felt-sense quality is of the tender mother love - a superradiant substance that unifies matter. Yet, it is a matter in a liquid that contains all elements, all levels of consciousness at the same time. This paradoxical state is intense and intimate in specific combinations: both/and/all/ neither/none/ infinitesimal/ infinite ... Again, *Pure Breath of Love* is a non-rational, mapless, and eternal realization that culminates as a permanent union between body and love.

WAITING
POEM BY TOKO-PA

There is a good kind of waiting
which trusts the agents of fermentation.
There is a waiting
which knows that in pulling away
one can more wholly return.
There is the waiting
which prepares oneself,
which anoints and adorns
and makes oneself plump
with readiness for love's return.
There is a good kind of waiting
which doesn't put oneself on hold
but rather adds layers to the grandness
of one's being worthy.
This sweet waiting
for one's fruits to ripen
doesn't stumble over itself
to be the first to give
but waits for the giving
to issue at its own graceful pace.

HEART OF PRAJNAPARAMITA SUTRA

Body is nothing more than emptiness,
emptiness is nothing more than body.
The body is exactly empty,
and emptiness is exactly body.
The other four aspects of human existence
- feeling, thought, will, and consciousness -
are likewise nothing more than emptiness,
and emptiness nothing more than they.
All things are empty:
Nothing is born, nothing dies,
nothing is pure, nothing is stained,
nothing increases and nothing decreases.
So, in emptiness, there is no body,
no feeling, no thought,
no will, no consciousness.
There are no eyes, no ears,
no nose, no tongue,
no body, no mind.
There is no seeing, no hearing,
no smelling, no tasting,

no touching, no imagining.
There is nothing seen, nor heard,
nor smelled, nor tasted,
nor touched, nor imagined.
There is no ignorance,
and no end to ignorance.
There is no old age and death,
and no end to old age and death.
There is no suffering, no cause of suffering,
no end to suffering, no path to follow.
There is no attainment of wisdom,
and no wisdom to attain.
The Bodhisattvas rely on the Perfection of Wisdom,
and so with no delusions,
they feel no fear,
and have Nirvana here and now.
All the Buddhas,
past, present, and future,
rely on the Perfection of Wisdom,
and live in full enlightenment.
The Perfection of Wisdom is the greatest mantra.
It is the clearest mantra,
the highest mantra,
the mantra that removes all suffering.
This is truth that cannot be doubted.
Say it so: Gone, gone, gone over, gone fully
    over. Awakened! So be it!

ABOUT THE AUTHOR

Charles Ridley began his studies in 1973 after he received one cranial session that expanded his consciousness for 30 days. He realized right then that cranial work would be his life's work. Charles experienced first-hand that cranial practice is a spiritual path that evolves consciousness. His cranial teacher, Dr. DeJarnette was Dr. Sutherland's student, and he directly transmitted Sutherland's essence in the cranial classes he taught.

Charles practiced biomechanical and functional cranial work for twenty of his forty-six years of cranial study and practice. Then, biodynamics spontaneously awakened in him in the mid 1990's. His inner experiences and meditations inspired Charles to write notes for his Biodynamic Cranial Touch Mentor Course that eventually became the book *Stillness*. Charles sat in stillness in the early mornings while filled with an ardent desire to receive the essence of Dr. Sutherland's transmission; he would write down what inwardly came to him.

Charles periodically exchanged sessions with three biodynamic cranial osteopaths. During one pivotal session in 1998 a biodynamic osteopath and teacher for Dr. James Jealous was giving Charles a session. Mid-session the DO blurted "Charles I'm panicking right now; I don't know what's going on or what to do!" Charles could sense that they were both basking in the vast radiance of long tide, and the DO's ego was recoiling due to fear of the unknown. Charles suggested the osteopath orient her awareness inward without expectations and sense what was arising. She relaxed and opened to her overpowering encounter. As the session continued Charles enjoyed contact with his inner Divine Child.

That experience during a session sealed the need for a book like *Stillness*: regardless of one's cranial background, sometimes the overwhelming power of an encounter with the Breath of Life can challenge any practitioner. He knew that the written word when based on direct inner body-felt experience acts like an oral transmission that supports a practitioner in being fully present to their encounters with the potency of the Breath of Life.

Charles is a semi-retired resident of Mexico, living in Puerto Vallarta. He writes, offers Private Intensives, and teaches post-biodynamic *Stillness Touch* graduate courses in Europe.

AFTERWORD

Material for this book is from 2002 to 2008; the subsequent years were spent clarifying the articulation to match a practitioner's inner experiences.

Chapter 1: The *pre-biodynamic* and *biodynamic* sections are from a Harbin Hot Springs *Initiatory Course* in 2005; the *post-biodynamic* section is from *Stillness* Chapter 9, which originated during an Ithaca, NY *Mentor Course* in 2003.

Chapter 2: Modified from the article *Body is Consciousness*, 2006.

Chapter 3: Modified from the blog, *Death of Biodynamics*, 2008.

Chapter 4: Modified from *Stillness Practices* Practitioner eBook, 2006.

Chapter 5: Modified from *Stillness Practices* eBook, 2006; Masculine and Feminine principles were compiled during a Muir Beach, CA *Mentor* in 2008.

Chapter 6-7: Modified from the article *Owning Your Grail Wound*, 2007.

Chapter 8: Comes from the Ithaca *Mentor Course* in 2003, the *Stillness Touch* Lay eBook 2010, and the *Stillness Touch* eBook, 2007.

Chapter 9: The *pre-biodynamic* and *biodynamic* sections are from a Harbin *Initiatory Course* 2005; the *post-biodynamic section* is from the Ithaca Mentor Course 2003, which became Chapter 9 of *Stillness, 2006.*

Appendix 1: An edited student presentation of a *Stillness Touch Lay Class* 2007.

Appendix 2: Edited from *Stillness Practices* for Practitioners eBook 2006.

Appendix 3: Quotes compiled over the years.

Appendix 4-5: Created by students during a Woodacre, CA *Mentor Course* 2006.

RECOMMENDED BOOKS AND RESOURCES

To purchase the following recommended books, please google the titles:

- *Gene Keys: Unlocking The Higher Purpose Hidden In Your DNA*. Richard Rudd, (2009). Gene Keys Publishing.
- *Meditations on the Tarot*. Anon, (2020) Angelico Press.
- *Tao of Leadership*. John Heider, (2006) Green Dragon Publishing.
- *Timeless Way of Building*. Christopher Alexander, (1979) Oxford University Press.
- *The Nature of Order: An Essay on the Art of Building and the Nature of the Universe*. Christopher Alexander, Four Volumes, (2004).
- *The Radiance Sutras*, Loren Roch (2014) Sounds True.
- *The White Hot Yoga of the Heart*. Saniel Bonder, (1995) Mt. Tam Empowerments.

To read the blog, articles, and eBooks or download the charts that formed this book, and to purchase Mp3 Meditations, Books, or enroll in Charles Ridley's classes visit:

http://www.DynamicStillness.com

BIBLIOGRAPHY

Aurobindo, S. (2018). *Sri Aurobindo or The Adventure of Consciousness* by Satpurim. Discovery Press.

Aurobindo, S.(1990). *The Synthesis of Yoga. The Path of the Heart for Spiritual Realization.* Lotus Press.

Becker, R. (2000). *The Stillness of Life.* Cambridge MA: Rudra Press.

Becker, R. (1997). *Life in Motion.* Cambridge MA: Rudra Press.

Becker, R. E. (1963). *Diagnostic Touch: Its principles and Application, Part I. Year Book of Selected Osteopathic Papers.*

Becker, R. E. (1964). *Diagnostic Touch: Its principles and Application, Part II* and III. *Year Book of Selected Osteopathic Papers.*

Becker, R. E. (1965). *Diagnostic Touch: Its principles and application, Part IV. Year Book of Selected Osteopathic Papers, Vol 2.*

Becker, R. O. (1990). *Cross Currents.* New York: Penguin Group Inc.

Bell, R. (2006). *Developmental Biology*. Paper presented at the Course Notes.

Blechschmidt & Gasser. (1978). *Biokinetics and Biodynamics of Human Differentiation*. Springfield, Illinois: Charles C. Thomas.

Blechschmidt, Erich (1970). *The Beginnings of Human Life*. New York: Springer.

Blechschmidt, Erich (2004). *The Ontogenetic Basis of Human Anatomy*. Berkeley: North Atlantic Books.

Blechschmidt, Erich (1961). *The Stages of Human Development Before Birth*. Philadelphia: W. B. Saunders.

Bonder, Saniel (2004). *Great Relief*. San Rafael, CA: Mt. Tam Awakenings.

Bonder, Saniel (1998). *Waking Down*. San Rafael, CA: Mt. Tam Awakenings.

Brooksby, R. (2005). *Be Still and Know* (4th Edition ed.). Lincoln, NE: iUniverse.

Chetanananda, Swami *Dynamic Stillness*. Two Volumes. Cambridge, MA: Rudra Press, 1990.

Cisler, T. (Ed.). (2003). *Are We On The Path? The Collected Works of Robert C. Fulford*. Indianapolis: The Cranial Academy.

Comeaux, Z. (2002). *Robert Fulford, D.O. and the Philosopher Physician*. Seattle: Eastland Press.

Dove, C. (2004). *Towards a New Theory*. Paper presented at the SCC Rollin Becker Memorial Lecture.

Duval, J. A. (2004). *Techniques Ostoépathiques d'Équilibre et d'Échanges Réciproques*. Vannes Cedex, France: Editions Sully.

Feely, R. A. (Ed.). (1988). *Clinical Cranial Osteopathy*. Indianapolis, Indiana: The Cranial Academy.

Frymann, V. (1998). *The Collected Papers of Viola M. Frymann, DO*. Indianapolis: American Academy of Osteopathy.

Handoll, N. (2000). *Anatomy of Potency*. Hereford, England: Osteopathic Supplies.

Jung, Carl Gustav (1996). *The Psychology of Kundalini Yoga*. Princeton, NJ: Princeton University Press.

Larre, Claude and Elisabeth Rochat de la Vallee (1995). *Rooted in Spirit: The Heart of Chinese Medicine*. Barrytown, NY: Station Hill Press.

Lee, R. P. (2005). *Interface: Mechanisms of Spirit in Osteopathy*. Portland, Oregon: Stillness Press.

Liem, T. (2004). *Cranial Osteopathy Principles and Practice*. London: Elsevier, Churchill Livingstone.

Magoun, H. I. (Ed.), (1951). *Osteopathy in the Cranial Field* (Original Edition ed.). Denver, Colorado: Sutherland Cranial Teaching Foundation.

Paulus, S. (2006). *The Osteopathic Experience of Fulcrums and the Emergence of Stillness*. In T. Liem (Ed.), *Morphodyunamik in der Osteopathie* (pp. 195-201). Stuttgart: Hippokrates Verlag.

Pischinger, Alfred (1991). *Matrix and Matrix Regulation: Basis for a Holistic Theory in Medicine*. Brussels: Haug International

Ridley, C. (2006). *Stillness*. Berkeley: North Atlantic Books.

Rudd, R. (2009). *Gene Keys: Unlocking The Higher Purpose Hidden In Your DNA*. Gene Keys Publishing

Russell, W. (1926). *The Universal ONE* (Vol. Volume 1). Waynesboro, Virginia: University of Science and Philosophy.

Russell, W. (1947). *The Secret of Light*. Waynesboro, Virginia: University of Science and Philosophy.

Russell, W. (1971). *The Message of the Divine Iliad, Vol. 1.* Virginia: University of Science and Philosophy.

Russell, W. (2006). *Gravitation and Radiation.* From www.walter-russell.com

Schooley, T. (1953). *The Fulcrum. 1953 OCA Journal,* 31.

Smith, F. (1990). *Inner Bridges.* Atlanta, Georgia: Humanics Limited.

Still, A., T. (1899). *Philosophy of Osteopathy.* Kirksville, Missouri.

Still, A., T. (1902). Untitled. *Journal of Osteopathy* (August), 275-277.

Still, A. T. (1902). *The Philosophy and Mechanical Principles of Osteopathy.* Kansas City: Hudson Kimberly Pub. Co.

Still, A. T. (1908). *Autobiography of A. T. Still* (5th Reprint ed.). Indianapolis: American Academy of Osteopathy.

Still, A. T. (1910). *Osteopathy, Research and Practice.* Seattle: Eastland Press.

Still, A. T. (1986). *The Philosophy and Mechanical Principles of Osteopathy.* Kirksville: Osteopathic Enterprise.

Still. A.T. (1991). *Early Osteopathy in the Words of A.T. Still.* Truman University Press.

Still, A. T. (2000). *Autobiography of A. T. Still* (5th Reprint ed.). Indianapolis: American Academy of Osteopathy.

Sutherland, A. (1962). *With Thinking Fingers.* Fort Worth, Texas: The Cranial Academy.

Sutherland, W.G. (1946). *Cranial Bowl* (second ed.) Fort Worth, Texas: Sutherland Cranial Teaching Foundation.

Sutherland, W.G. (1998). *Contributions of Thought - The Collected Writings of William Garner Sutherland, D.O.* (second ed.). Fort Worth, Texas

Sutherland, W. G. (1990). *Teachings in the Science of Osteopathy.* Rudra Press.

Swedenborg, E. (1899). *On Tremulation* (Reprinted in 1976 ed.). Boston: Massachusetts New-Church Union.

Swedenborg, E. (1918). *Economy of the Animal Kingdom, III The Fibre.* Philadelphia: Swedenborg Scientific Association.

Taylor, D. (2008). *The Concept of the Fulcrum.* Thesis. Canadian College of Osteopathy.

Wales, A. (1953). *The Management, Reactions and Systemic Effects of Fluctuation of the Cerebrospinal Fluid. 1953 OAC Journal,* 39.

Wales, A. (1986). *The Still Point.* Cranial Academy Newsletter, *39*, 1-2.

Wernham, J. (1995). *Lectures on Osteopathy.* Maidstone, Kent: Maidstone College of Osteopathy.

Wernham, J. (1999a). *Classical Osteopathy.* Maidstone, Kent: John Werham College.

Wernham, J. (1999b). *The Life and Times of Martin Littlejohn.* Maidstone, Kent: John Wernham College.

Wernham, J. (2003). *Lectures on Osteopathy.* Maidstone, Kent: John Wernham College.

ENDNOTES

1. Sutherland, W.G. (1998). *Contributions of Thought - The Collected Writings of William Garner Sutherland, D.O.* (second ed.). Fort Worth, Texas. 188.

2. Ibid. 254.

3. *Dynamic Stillness Volume 1 & 2.* (1990) Rudra Press. and see Kashmir Shaivism in Appendix 1.

4. Sutherland, W.G. (1946) *Cranial Bowl* (second ed.)Fort Worth, Texas: Sutherland Cranial Teaching Foundation. Preface.

5. *The Heart Sutra of Prajnaparamita* http://webspace.ship.edu/cgboer/heartsutra.html

6. See Chapter 2 *Orienting to Anatomy is Not Neutral* and Chapter 3 *Practitioner Recoils.*

7. Click the links below for the photos of the Sutherlands headstones:
https://www.findagrave.com/memorial/104402276/william-g-sutherland/

https://www.findagrave.com/memorial/108878802/adah-sutherland/

8. See Figure 2 below.

9. This is characterized in Ridley, C. (2006) *Stillness*. Chapter 9.

10. *Stillness* Chapter 9 introduced this enfoldment as *Pure Breath of Life*, but the name has since changed to *Pure Breath of Love* because the inner body-felt quality is like the Breath of the Tender Mother Love.

11. See Appendix 1.

12. Jung, C.G. (2009) *Red Book: Libre Novus*. W.W Norton & Co. 346.

13. We will explore the Core Erotic Wound in-depth in Chapters 6 and 7.

14. The recoils from love are detailed in Chapters 3 and 7.

15. *The Heart Sutra of Prajnaparamita.*

16. Marina Abramovic, (2016) *Walk Through Walls: A Memoir.* Crown Archetype.

17. Sutherland, W.G. (1980) *Teaching in the Science of Osteopathy.* Rudra Press. 167.

18. See Chapter 3, and the Appendix 6 Chart *Caregiver Vulnerabilities to Ethical Misconduct.*

19. See Chapter 3 *Practitioner Recoils that Impede Pure Breath of Love.*

20. See W.G. Sutherland in Appendix 3.

21. See Erich Blechschmidt's list of books in the Bibliography.

22. Jung, C. (1966) *The Psychology of Kundalini Yoga.* Princeton, NJ: Princeton University Press. 73.

23. See *Treatment Reactions* in the Appendix of *Stillness;* also for more on the descending current practices, see Chapter 6 *Owning Your Grail Wound.*

24. Read the Introduction, *Blechschmidt* in Chapter 2, *Eh in* Chapter 5, *Walter Russell* and *Emanuel Swedenborg* in Appendix 3. Also see *Wolff's Law* in Appendix 2 of *Stillness.*

25. See the Appendix 6 Chart, *Caregiver Vulnerabilities to Ethical Misconduct.*

26. See Rollin Becker in Appendix 3.

27. Sutherland, W. *Collected Writings.* (1967) Ed. Adah Sutherland and Anne L. Wales. Fort Worth, TX: Sutherland Cranial Teaching Foundation. 233-246.

28. See Chapters 6 & 7.

29. See Chapters 6 and 7, and the Appendix 6 Chart *Caregiver Vulnerabilities.*

30. For a list of the chakra functions, see eBook, Ridley, C (2000) *Beyond Stillness*, The Chakras.

31. See Chapters 6 and 7.

32. See Chapter 7, *The Core Erotic Wound and Our Unconscious Recoils from Love.*

33. Ridley, C. (2006) *Stillness: Biodynamic Cranial Practice and the Evolution of Consciousness.* 32.

34. See Chapters 6 and 7.

35. Hermes Trismegistus *Tabula Smaragdina - The Emerald Table*, translated into English by Robert Steele & Dorothy W. Singer, *Proceedings of the Royal Society of Medicine*, XXI, 1928, 42.

36. Rudd, R. (2009) *Gene Keys:Unlocking The Higher Purpose Hidden In Your DNA.* Gene Keys Pub.

37. Douglas-Klotz, N. (1999) *The Hidden Gospel.* Quest Books. Chapter 3.

38. See Carl Jung in Appendix 3.

39. Read Segal, S. (1996) *Collision With The Infinite: A Life Beyond the Personal Self.* Blue Dove Press

40. See Chapters 6 and 7.

41. *Sri Aurobindo or The Adventure of Consciousness* by Satpurim. (2018) Discovery Publishers https://kfireforall.tumblr.-com/post/186743813610/the-higher-one-rises-the-farther-one-is-pulled

42. Brown, B. Quotes https://www.goodreads.com/author/quotes/162578.Bren_Brown

43. For more information, Google, *"Hermes Caduceus"* and see the Appendix 6 Chart *Caregiver Vulnerabilities to Ethical Misconduct.*

44. See Ridley, C. (2000) eBook *Stillness Practices.* Chapter 2.

45. To read Rudolf Steiner's characterization of Luciferic qualities Google *"Lucifer Waldorf Watch"*

46. Google, *"Seifritz on Protoplasm - Full Film"* to see the slime mold film on Youtube.

47. *Letters from Sri Ramanasramam.* (2006) by Sr Ramanasramam Tiruvannamalai/India. Letter 80.

48. See Ridley, C. (2006) *Stillness* Chapter 9.

49. See Chapter 4 *Transmute the Shadow - Dissolve the Inner War.*

50. See Chapter 3 Figure 3 *Practitioner Recoils that Impede Pure Breath of Love*

51. See Chapter 8, *The Inner Qualities of Enfleshment.*

52. If a detailed somatic navigation can help you integrate aspects of the *Core Wound*: read *Stillness Practices* Chapters 1 and 4, available in English, French, and German - in the Dynamic-Stillness.com Store.

53. You can download the charts from DynamicStillness.com "News and Events."

54. See the Appendix 6 Chart *Caregiver Vulnerabilities to Ethical Misconduct.*

55. To gain an appreciation of this process, review Figures 8, 9, 10.

56. See Abrams, D. (1996) *The Spell of the Sensuous.* New York: Pantheon.

57. *Love Itself.* A song by Leonard Cohen.

58. *The Science of Soul* (1977) Shree Swami Vyas Dev Ji Maharaj, Yoga Niketan. 35.

59. *Enlightenment of the Whole Body* (1974) Bubba Free John, Dawn Horse Press. 400.

60. *Dynamic Stillness* Volume 1, (1990) Swami Chetanananda, Rudra Press. 74-75.

61. Larre, C (1995) *Rooted in Spirit: The Heart of Chinese Medicine.* Barrytown, NY. Station Hill Press.

62. Adams, R. (1995) *The Collected Works of Robert Adams.* E-book-version. 1489.

63. Detailed book and article references are in the Bibliography; particularly see Taylor, D.

64. Inspired by Ridley, C. (2006) *Stillness,* Chapters 5-10.

www.ingramcontent.com/pod-product-compliance
Lightning Source LLC
Chambersburg PA
CBHW060312030426
42336CB00011B/1013